Kriya Yoga

A Guide to Awaken the Chakras and Kundalini

(The Scientific Process of Soul Culture and the Essence of All Religions)

James Nicoletti

Published By **Simon Dough**

James Nicoletti

All Rights Reserved

Kriya Yoga: A Guide to Awaken the Chakras and Kundalini (The Scientific Process of Soul Culture and the Essence of All Religions)

ISBN   978-1-9990225-7-0

No part of this guidebook shall be reproduced in any form without permission in writing from the publisher except in the case of brief quotations embodied in critical articles or reviews.

Legal & Disclaimer

Table Of Contents

Chapter 1: The Fundamentals Of Kriya Yoga

Pranayama: The Science of Breath Control

In the historical expertise of yoga, the exercise of pranayama holds a completely unique vicinity. Prana, regularly referred to as the lifestyles strain power, is the vital energy that animates all dwelling beings. The word 'pranayama' is derived from Sanskrit phrases: 'prana' this means that life pressure, and 'ayama' which means that manage or expansion. Therefore, pranayama can be understood due to the fact the era of breath manipulate or the growth of existence pressure energy.

Pranayama is an essential part of Kriya Yoga, a non secular direction that leads the seeker inside the direction of self-popularity. While Kriya Yoga encompasses numerous practices, pranayama is taken into consideration fundamental and important. It is thru the exercise of pranayama that we gain mastery over our breath, which in flip allows us modify our physical, intellectual, and emotional states.

The breath is not truely a bodily gadget; it's miles the bridge that connects the frame, thoughts, and soul. By consciously controlling and directing the breath, we will have an effect on and harmonize the ones elements of our being. Through ordinary workout, pranayama allows us to purify the electricity channels in our frame and decorate the drift of prana, main to superior health and power.

Apart from its physical benefits, pranayama has a profound effect at the mind. The mind is frequently careworn, whole of incessant mind and distractions. Through the exercising of pranayama, we discover ways to quiet the mind and domesticate inner stillness. This allows us to delve deeper into meditation and enjoy moments of heightened popularity and non secular connection.

Pranayama practices variety of their techniques and complexities, starting from easy diaphragmatic respiration to superior practices like trade nostril respiration and breath retention. However, it's miles crucial to method pranayama with steering and recognize for its capability strength. The breath is a touchy and powerful tool, and its manipulation ought to be completed with recognition and sensitivity.

For seekers of Kriya Yoga, pranayama serves as a gateway to self-interest. It is a effective device that allows the awakening of our dormant non secular potential and enables us transcend the rules of the physical body and the ego. Through the regular practice of pranayama, we are capable of steadily unfastened up the hidden geographical regions of our being and embark on a transformative journey towards self-discovery and enlightenment.

In end, pranayama is a profound era that offers a large number of benefits for without a doubt everybody, regardless of their non secular direction or statistics. Whether you're a pro yogi or simply beginning your adventure in the route of self-attention, the exercise of pranayama can be a treasured tool for harmonizing the frame, mind, and soul. As you delve into the depths of breath manage, be prepared to loose up the hidden functionality internal yourself and enjoy the transformative energy of pranayama.

Asanas: Physical Postures for Balance and Alignment

Asanas: Physical Postures for Balance and Alignment

In the arena of Kriya Yoga, the exercise of asanas holds big importance as they function gateways to attain balance and alignment in each the physical and active our our bodies. Asanas, or physical postures, are not simplest a way to gain flexibility and strength but additionally a pathway inside the course of self-popularity and spiritual increase. Whether you're an professional yogi or a beginner at the direction of Kriya Yoga, expertise and incorporating asanas into your exercise can bring about profound variations.

The asanas in Kriya Yoga are designed to harmonize the body, mind, and spirit. They purpose to create a rustic of equilibrium via aligning the bodily frame's electricity centers, or chakras, which might be essential for common properly-being. Through ordinary practice, those postures help release any blockages or stagnant strength, allowing the lifestyles pressure, or prana, to float freely at some level in the body.

One of the essential components of asanas in Kriya Yoga is the point of interest on right alignment. By aligning the frame correctly, you could simply enjoy the proper essence and advantages of every posture. Proper alignment now not handiest prevents injuries however additionally ensures that the energy channels, or nadis, are unobstructed, facilitating the clean flow into of prana.

Each asana in Kriya Yoga has a particular motive and effect at the body and thoughts.

Some postures, together with the Mountain Pose (Tadasana), domesticate stability and grounding, on the same time as others, which encompass the Tree Pose (Vrikshasana), sell stability and focus. The exercise of asanas additionally cultivates mindfulness and self-interest, as practitioners are recommended to be truly discovered in every posture, looking at their breath and bodily sensations.

It is essential to have a observe that the workout of asanas in Kriya Yoga isn't restricted to bodily workout; it is a manner to move past the physical and connect to the deeper elements of our being. The postures function gadget to put together the frame for meditation and inner exploration. They assist in calming the thoughts, freeing tension, and getting equipped the body to sit down simply for prolonged durations of time in meditation.

Whether you're trying to find bodily health, emotional balance, or religious boom, incorporating the workout of asanas to your Kriya Yoga adventure can be immensely beneficial. As you delve deeper into this ancient exercise, keep in thoughts to approach every posture with mindfulness, staying power, and reverence. Allow the asanas to guide you toward self-popularity and a deeper expertise of your proper nature. Embrace the transformative power of asanas and embark on a journey of balance, alignment, and self-discovery.

Meditation Techniques in Kriya Yoga

Meditation is a powerful device that allows us to connect with our internal selves, discover peace, and revel in self-interest. In the arena of Kriya Yoga, meditation holds a special vicinity because it paperwork the center of this religious workout. Through numerous meditation techniques, Kriya Yoga practitioners can embark on a transformative adventure toward self-awareness and internal bliss.

One of the vital meditation techniques in Kriya Yoga is the workout of breath control. Known as pranayama, this technique includes regulating and controlling the breath to calm the thoughts and wake up dormant spiritual energies interior. By focusing on the inhalation and exhalation, practitioners can enter a country of deep rest and heightened attention. This method allows in purifying the thoughts, body, and spirit, getting prepared them for deeper ranges of meditation.

Another vital meditation method in Kriya Yoga is the exercising of mantra repetition. Mantras are sacred sounds or phrases which can be repeated silently or aloud during meditation. These mantras deliver effective vibrations that help quiet the thoughts and bring about a kingdom of harmony and inner peace. Through the repetition of mantras, practitioners can go past their ordinary cognizance and get right of entry to better geographical regions of consciousness, bringing them toward self-recognition.

Visualization is however a few different meditation method utilized in Kriya Yoga. By visualizing particular snap shots or symbols within the direction of meditation, practitioners can harness the power of the mind to take vicinity their dreams and hook up with higher non secular energies. This approach permits in developing more interest, recognition, and clarity of idea, allowing people to faucet into their internal capacity and appear notable modifications of their lives.

In Kriya Yoga, the workout of meditation additionally includes experiencing the internal silence. By withdrawing the senses from out of doors distractions, practitioners can turn their interest inward and revel in the profound stillness that exists inner. This approach permits for a deep reference to the divine and allows the awakening of spiritual popularity.

No do not forget who you're or what your history may be, the meditation techniques in Kriya Yoga provide a route within the route of self-interest and internal transformation. Whether you are a newbie or a complicated practitioner, the ones techniques can be tailor-made to fit your individual dreams and talents. By incorporating the ones techniques into your every day regular, you may experience the profound benefits of Kriya Yoga and embark on a adventure closer to self-discovery and internal bliss.

Mantra Chanting: Harnessing the Power of Sound

In the sector of non secular practices, mantra chanting holds a totally specific place. It is a powerful tool that lets in us to tap into the transformative energy of sound vibrations and connect to our inner selves. In the ancient exercise of Kriya Yoga, mantra chanting performs a pivotal function in the adventure inside the course of self-cognizance.

Mantras, regularly seemed as sacred syllables or phrases, have been used for masses of years during numerous cultures and traditions. They own the functionality to create a profound effect on our bodily, intellectual, and non secular properly-being. The vibrations generated by way of using chanting mantras resonate inside our being, selling deep rest, heightened popularity, and spiritual awakening.

The practice of mantra chanting in Kriya Yoga involves the repetition of precise sounds or phrases which might be carefully decided on to align with the seeker's motive and non secular course. These mantras act as a bridge among the individual and the divine, deliberating a deeper connection and a channeling of divine energy. By repeating those mantras with reputation and devotion, the seeker can get right of entry to higher states of popularity and enjoy a experience of concord with the divine.

The strength of mantra chanting lies no longer simplest inside the terms themselves but additionally within the aim and power behind them. When we chant a mantra with sincerity and reverence, we infuse it with our private unique vibrations, magnifying its efficiency. This technique facilitates to purify our thoughts and emotions, growing a immoderate wonderful and harmonious internal surroundings.

Moreover, clinical research has set up that mantra chanting has a profound impact on our thoughts and worried device. It has been determined to reduce pressure, enhance cognitive feature, and enhance regular well-being. The repetitive nature of chanting induces a meditative country, calming the thoughts and selling a experience of internal peace.

For the ones at the course of Kriya Yoga, mantra chanting is an essential exercise. It not only aids in deepening meditation however moreover serves as a powerful tool for self-transformation. Through constant repetition of mantras, the seeker can cultivate inner region, attention, and religious boom.

Chapter 2: The Eight Limbs

Yama: Ethical Guidelines for a Harmonious Life

In the historical teachings of Kriya Yoga, Yama is appeared as one of the essential pillars for essential a existence of concord and self-awareness. Yama can be understood as a difficult and fast of ethical tips that help people cultivate a balanced and virtuous existence. These necessities are not unique to those running towards Kriya Yoga; they may be applicable and applicable to anyone trying to find a enormous and sensible existence.

Yama encompasses 5 mind, every representing a precious element of ethical conduct. The first principle is Ahimsa, which interprets to non-violence or non-harming. It encourages humans to increase compassion and kindness to all dwelling beings, fostering a feel of harmony and interconnectedness. By schooling Ahimsa, we discover ways to deal with ourselves and others with respect, maintaining off moves that purpose harm or suffering.

The 2d principle is Satya, meaning truthfulness. Satya encourages humans to be sincere of their mind, phrases, and actions. By embracing truthfulness, we create an environment of accept as real with and authenticity, every inner ourselves and in our relationships. Satya teaches us to align our intentions with our moves, fostering integrity and readability of reason.

The 0.33 principle is Asteya, which interprets to non-stealing. Asteya encourages humans to chorus from taking what isn't rightfully theirs, both in cloth possessions and within the intangible additives of existence, together with time, strength, or interest. By practising Asteya, we domesticate a revel in of contentment and gratitude for what we've, putting off the want for excessive acquisition or exploitation.

The fourth principle is Brahmacharya, frequently interpreted as moderation or celibacy. Brahmacharya encourages people to channel their energy and goals in a balanced way, fending off immoderate indulgence or attachment. By schooling Brahmacharya, we learn how to harness our crucial energy and direct it toward our spiritual increase and self-recognition.

The fifth and very last precept of Yama is Aparigraha, meaning non-possessiveness or non-greediness. Aparigraha encourages people to detach themselves from cloth possessions and keep away from immoderate attachment. By working toward Aparigraha, we unfastened ourselves from the burdens of greed, jealousy, and possessiveness, allowing us to embody a existence of simplicity, contentment, and internal abundance.

By incorporating these moral pointers into our every day lives, we will create a harmonious and balanced lifestyles. The standards of Yama provide a roadmap for navigating our interactions with ourselves, others, and the arena spherical us. Regardless of our religious route or personal ideals, those ideas keep sizeable fee in guiding us closer to a existence of compassion, integrity, and self-interest.

In quit, Yama serves as a transformative device for human beings searching out to manual a useful and giant lifestyles. By embracing the thoughts of non-violence, truthfulness, non-stealing, moderation, and non-possessiveness, we are capable of domesticate a harmonious lifestyles and make contributions to the properly-being of ourselves and the area at massive. Yama isn't constrained to the exercising of Kriya Yoga; it is a ordinary manual for every person on the direction within the path of self-focus and achievement.

Niyama: Personal Observances for Self-Discipline

Niyama: Personal Observances for Self-Discipline

In the path of self-awareness and non secular increase, place plays a important characteristic. It is thru challenge that we cultivate strength of will, make bigger inner strength, and acquire a country of harmony inside ourselves and with the sector round us. Niyama, one of the 8 limbs of Kriya Yoga, offers practical suggestions for non-public observances that facilitate energy of will and lead us within the path of self-reputation.

Niyama consists of five vital practices which may be aimed toward nurturing our internal being and growing a exquisite environment for non secular improvement. These practices are:

1. Saucha (Purity): Saucha includes retaining bodily, highbrow, and emotional purity. It encourages us to keep our our our bodies clean, eat nourishing food, and interact in sports that sell highbrow clarity and emotional well-being. By operating toward saucha, we create a harmonious basis for non secular boom.

2. Santosha (Contentment): Santosha is the exercise of cultivating contentment and gratitude. It teaches us to locate joy and pride inside the gift 2nd, in preference to constantly in search of out of doors validation or fabric possessions. Santosha enables us extend a revel in of internal peace and reduces the distractions that save you religious development.

3. Tapas (Discipline): Tapas refers to the exercise of power of will and austerity. It encourages us to conquer our goals, amplify energy of thoughts, and have interaction in practices that challenge our consolation zones. Tapas allows us construct internal energy and resilience, permitting us to navigate lifestyles's challenges with grace and backbone.

four. Svadhyaya (Self-Study): Svadhyaya consists of the observe of religious texts, introspection, and self-mirrored picture. It encourages us to delve deep into our inner selves, understand our mind and feelings, and gain insights into our real nature. Svadhyaya lets in us increase self-awareness and a deeper statistics of the spiritual route.

five. Ishvara Pranidhana (Surrender to the Divine): Ishvara Pranidhana is the exercise of surrendering to a better electricity or the divine. It includes letting bypass of our ego and trusting in a extra intelligence that publications us in the path of our most capability. By surrendering to the divine, we domesticate humility, popularity, and faith, which can be vital for religious growth.

Incorporating those practices into our each day lives can extensively decorate our journey towards self-popularity. Whether you're a novice or an skilled practitioner of Kriya Yoga, embracing the personal observances of niyama can bring about profound adjustments for your existence. They provide a roadmap for energy of will, internal growth, and the belief of our actual nature.

Remember, the ones practices are not intended to be rigid guidelines however instead mild recommendations that encourage us to cultivate excessive high-quality habits and attitudes. By embracing niyama, we can cultivate strength of will, purify our minds and our our bodies, and create a solid basis for non secular growth. So, embark in this transformative journey and enjoy the profound advantages of niyama to your lifestyles.

Asana: Cultivating Physical and Mental Stability

In the historical exercise of Kriya Yoga, one of the essential elements is the cultivation of physical and intellectual balance thru the workout of asanas. Asanas, or yoga postures, are not simply bodily sports but a technique of harmonizing the body and mind, paving the way for self-focus.

For every body, no matter their information or degree of revel in, asanas offer a path to discover stability and balance in each the physical and mental nation-states. Through the workout of asanas, we learn how to growth popularity of our physical body, its boundaries, and its ability. As we have interaction in each posture, we recognition on our breath, searching at the sensations that rise up, and cultivating a deep connection between the body, breath, and mind.

The exercise of asanas in Kriya Yoga goes past the physical advantages. It acts as a stepping stone inside the route of self-interest via manner of way of fostering attention, trouble, and intellectual clarity. Each asana not simplest stretches and strengthens the body but additionally brings interest to the prevailing 2d, growing a rustic of mindfulness and internal stillness.

In the adventure of Kriya Yoga, asanas function a tool to purify the body and prepare it for the better degrees of meditation. By schooling asanas often, we release bodily and intellectual anxiety, beautify flexibility, and decorate commonplace nicely-being. This physical and intellectual balance becomes the muse upon which we're capable of assemble a deeper statistics of ourselves and our connection to the area.

Whether you're a amateur or a seasoned practitioner, the workout of asanas in Kriya Yoga offers huge advantages. It allows you to music inwards, grow to be aware about your body, and find out the profound outcomes of integrating body and thoughts. Through ordinary exercise, you may observe expanded power, flexibility, and focus, every on and stale the mat.

In quit, asanas are an crucial a part of the Kriya Yoga lifestyle, serving as a manner to cultivate physical and intellectual balance. By appealing in the exercise of asanas, we discover ways to harmonize our body and mind, paving the manner for self-interest. Regardless of your degree of enjoy or information, asanas offer a path to discover balance, boom cognizance, and decorate regular properly-being. Embrace the exercise of asanas and embark on a journey toward self-discovery and inner transformation through the beautiful course of Kriya Yoga.

Pranayama: Expanding Vital Energy through Breathwork

Pranayama: Expanding Vital Energy thru Breathwork

In the ancient yogic lifestyle, the workout of Pranayama has been respected as a effective device for harnessing and increasing critical energy. Prana, often called the life strain or crucial energy, is taken into consideration the essence that sustains all living beings. Pranayama, which translates to "extension of the lifestyles stress," is a workout that specializes in controlling and directing the breath to beautify the go with the flow of prana in the body.

Pranayama is an vital part of the transformative and profound machine known as Kriya Yoga. Kriya Yoga, a route toward self-awareness, combines numerous yogic techniques, which includes asanas (postures), meditation, and breathwork, to awaken the dormant spiritual energy internal every seeker. Through the practice of Pranayama, feasible faucet into this massive reservoir of prana, principal to accelerated energy, highbrow readability, and non secular boom.

The breath is not merely a physical method; it's miles a bridge connecting the frame, mind, and spirit. By consciously regulating the breath, one profits mastery over the mind and feelings, deliberating a deeper connection to the divine indoors. Breath manipulate techniques in Pranayama involve precise styles of inhalation, exhalation, and retention, with the reason of purifying and balancing the subtle electricity channels (nadis) in the frame.

Regular exercise of Pranayama has severa benefits for practitioners of Kriya Yoga and all and sundry attempting to find to enhance their properly-being. It will increase lung functionality, improves respiration characteristic, and oxygenates the blood, leading to improved fashionable health. By calming the worried device, it reduces stress, tension, and horrible emotions, promoting intellectual and emotional stability.

Moreover, Pranayama acts as a catalyst for non secular awakening, because it opens the gateway to higher states of interest. As the breath will become touchy and the drift of prana harmonizes, practitioners may additionally moreover experience a profound revel in of inner peace, improved recognition, and a deep connection to the standard lifestyles strain.

To embark on the direction of Pranayama, it's far important to examine from an expert trainer who can manual you within the right techniques and make certain a consistent and powerful practice. As with any yogic problem, consistency and endurance are key. Begin with simple respiration sports activities, little by little increasing the duration and complexity as you development.

In give up, Pranayama is a powerful practice inside the realm of Kriya Yoga that allows individuals of all backgrounds to tap into the limitless reservoir of vital electricity inside. Whether you are looking for bodily properly-being, intellectual readability, or non secular boom, incorporating Pranayama into your every day everyday can result in transformative effects. Embrace the energy of your breath and permit it guide you on a profound adventure toward self-popularity and inner transformation.

Pratyahara: Mastering the Withdrawal of Senses

In the widespread realm of spiritual practices, Kriya Yoga stands proud as a profound course towards self-recognition. Rooted in historical information, Kriya Yoga gives a systematic approach to harmonizing the frame, mind, and spirit. One of the important factors of this transformative journey is the exercising of Pratyahara, the artwork of chickening out the senses.

Pratyahara, derived from the Sanskrit phrases "prati" because of this "inside the course of" and "ahara" which means "food" or "input," refers to the conscious withdrawal of interest from external stimuli. In a global bombarded with the useful resource of endless distractions, gaining knowledge of the withdrawal of senses is essential for deepening our non secular exercise and reclaiming our inner peace.

The exercising of Pratyahara lets in us to disconnect from the outside international, quieting the thoughts and turning our attention inward. By consciously taking flight our senses from the sensory inputs that constantly call for our hobby, we are capable of redirect our attention toward the subtle geographical regions of our being.

Through Pratyahara, we benefit manipulate over our senses and prevent them from dictating our mind, feelings, and actions. By disengaging from the outdoor stimuli, we growth a heightened hobby of our inner landscape, fostering introspection and self-mirrored image. This inward adventure opens the gateway to self-hobby, permitting us to connect with our proper essence and experience the profound depths of our being.

Pratyahara isn't always about renouncing the arena or shunning sensory research. Rather, it is an invitation to consciously pick out what we have interaction with and the way we reply to the stimuli spherical us. It empowers us to emerge as the masters of our senses in preference to being managed with the resource of them.

The exercise of Pratyahara can be cultivated through severa techniques, together with breath recognition, meditation, and mindfulness. By redirecting our interest to the breath, we anchor ourselves in the gift 2nd, untangling from the internet of beyond regrets and future troubles. Through meditation, we broaden the capacity to study our thoughts and feelings without getting entangled in them, cultivating a nation of equanimity and internal stillness.

Pratyahara is a essential step on the course of Kriya Yoga, allowing us to move beyond the policies of the outdoor worldwide and dive into the boundless ocean of our inner being. It is a exercising that can be protected into our each day lives, allowing us to navigate the place with readability, compassion, and inner strength.

In prevent, Pratyahara is a transformative exercising that empowers every seeker, regardless of their information or ideals, to grasp the withdrawal of senses. By consciously disconnecting from out of doors stimuli, we embark on a profound journey of self-discovery and self-recognition. Through the exercise of Pratyahara, we reclaim our internal peace, deepen our non secular connection, and unfastened up the huge ability within us. Embrace this beneficial exercise, and allow the beauty of Pratyahara manual you within the path of a lifestyles of fulfillment, cause, and self-cognizance.

Dharana: Focusing the Mind on a Single Point

In the historic knowledge of Kriya Yoga, one of the fundamental practices is Dharana, the art of focusing the thoughts on a unmarried component. Dharana, this means that that that attention, is a effective device that lets in us to gather deep stages of consciousness and internal stillness. Through this exercising, we will harness the first-rate capability of our thoughts and connect with our genuine nature.

In extremely-current speedy-paced worldwide, our minds are frequently scattered, continuously bombarded with distractions from all instructions. We locate ourselves multitasking, now not capable of pay hobby on one aspect at a time. This loss of attention can motive pressure, anxiety, and a enjoy of disconnection from ourselves and the arena round us. Dharana offers a technique to this modern seize 22 scenario thru training us a way to deliver our hobby back to the prevailing moment and domesticate a country of deep interest.

The workout of Dharana consists of deciding on a unmarried point of recognition and directing our hobby towards it. This element may be something – a physical object, a mantra, the breath, or even a visualization. By gently guiding our thoughts decrease returned up to now every time it wanders, we regularly educate our intellectual schools to emerge as extra disciplined and focused.

Through regular exercise, the blessings of Dharana come to be apparent. We experience an expanded capability to pay interest, stronger reminiscence, and advanced highbrow readability. Our mind will become more calm and balanced, permitting us to make better alternatives and navigate life's traumatic situations quite in reality. Additionally, Dharana opens the door to deeper states of meditation, in which we're capable of get proper of entry to better geographical areas of focus and enjoy profound religious insights.

Dharana isn't always confined to the meditation cushion; it can be practiced in any interest. Whether we are engaged in paintings, pastimes, or maybe mundane every day duties, we are able to comply with the requirements of Dharana to keep our whole interest to the prevailing second. By doing so, we infuse our moves with mindfulness and presence, major to more overall performance, creativity, and achievement.

In quit, Dharana is a transformative exercising which can benefit each person, irrespective of their non secular ancient beyond or ideals. It is a tool for cultivating reputation, readability, and internal stillness in a global packed with distractions. Through the workout of Dharana, we embark on a journey towards self-awareness, discovering our proper nature and connecting with the infinite capability inside us. Whether you're new to Kriya Yoga or a pro practitioner, embracing Dharana will truely beautify your religious adventure and convey profound immoderate high-quality modifications to your existence.

Dhyana: Deepening the State of Meditation

In the ancient practice of Kriya Yoga, one of the essential elements is the cultivation of Dhyana, which refers back to the deepening of the dominion of meditation. Dhyana lets in practitioners to transport beyond the ground diploma of recognition and revel in profound states of attention, major them in the direction of self-recognition.

For clearly absolutely everyone, irrespective of their records or non secular beliefs, Dhyana holds the ability to release the large reservoirs of internal peace, readability, and divine connection. Through regular exercise, humans can get right of access to a country of deep stillness, free from the distractions of the outdoor worldwide. It is on this profound stillness that you could honestly in reality connect with their innermost being.

The technique of deepening the nation of meditation starts offevolved with finding a quiet and snug region, free from out of doors disturbances. As the seeker settles into a comfortable posture, they regularly withdraw their senses from the out of doors environment, turning their interest inward. This turning inward is the first step toward Dhyana.

With centered hobby, the practitioner starts offevolved to have a have a look at the breath, the use of it as an anchor to normal the thoughts. As the mind turns into more settled, thoughts step by step subside, giving way to a kingdom of natural recognition. This is in which the proper essence of Dhyana lies - in the experience of herbal attention, indifferent from the fluctuations of the thoughts.

Through everyday workout, the nation of Dhyana turns into extra on hand and accessible. As the practitioner delves deeper into their meditation, they'll begin to revel in profound states of bliss, insights, and a heightened feel of interconnectedness with all of introduction. These research aren't limited to a pick few; they'll be to be had to every seeker of reality and self-awareness.

Dhyana isn't really restricted to the time spent in formal meditation; it could be protected into each aspect of existence. By bringing a meditative excellent to each day sports, humans can experience a deep experience of presence and mindfulness. This integration of Dhyana into every day life outcomes in a kingdom of non-forestall popularity, wherein each 2nd will become an possibility for growth and self-discovery.

In the journey of Kriya Yoga, Dhyana plays a important feature in unraveling the layers of illusion and unveiling the right nature of the self. It is through this deepening of the nation of meditation that seekers can in the end realise their interconnectedness with the universe and experience the profound delight and peace that lie internal.

Whether you're new to Kriya Yoga or were schooling for years, the exploration of Dhyana is an important trouble of the direction inside the path of self-interest. Embrace this practice with an open coronary coronary coronary heart and mind, and you could find out the transformative electricity of deepening the dominion of meditation for your personal life.

Samadhi: The Ultimate Union with the Divine

Samadhi: The Ultimate Union with the Divine

In the huge realm of religious practices, there exists a route that leads every seeker in the direction of the remaining aim of self-consciousness and union with the Divine. This route, known as Kriya Yoga, offers a profound and transformative journey for absolutely everyone who embark upon it. At the heart of this route lies the top of religious attainment - Samadhi, the final union with the Divine.

Samadhi can be described as a kingdom of entire absorption and oneness with the Divine recognition. It is a transcendent revel in in which the man or woman self merges with the famous Self, dissolving all obstacles and barriers. In this nation, one attains a profound sense of peace, bliss, and interconnectedness with all of creation.

The exercising of Kriya Yoga serves as a effective device to put together the seeker for the experience of Samadhi. Through a scientific approach that combines numerous techniques of breath control, meditation, and strength of will, Kriya Yoga cultivates the important capabilities of reputation, purity, and give up to facilitate the adventure towards Samadhi.

One of the important thing factors of Kriya Yoga is pranayama, the generation of breath manage. Through precise respiratory techniques, the practitioner harmonizes the glide of prana (existence strain electricity) inside the frame, purifying and revitalizing the entire tool. As the burdened mind will become calm and the frame relaxes, the seeker actions in the direction of the usa of Samadhi.

Meditation is a few exceptional crucial issue of Kriya Yoga, permitting the practitioner to delve deep into the geographical regions of cognizance. By retreating the senses and focusing the mind on a designated object of meditation, one grade by grade transcends the regulations of the bodily frame and reaches the location of pure cognizance. In this heightened country of recognition, the seeker starts offevolved to experience glimpses of Samadhi, paving the way for the very last union with the Divine.

The journey inside the direction of Samadhi requires energy of will, perseverance, and a deep longing for religious awakening. It is a route that transcends spiritual barriers and is open to certainly absolutely everyone who seeks to understand their actual nature. Whether you are a novice or an professional practitioner of Kriya Yoga, the route to

Samadhi gives a profound possibility for self-discovery and transformation.

In the pages of "Kriya Yoga: A Journey Towards Self-Realization for Every Seeker," you'll discover steering, insights, and realistic techniques that will help you navigate this sacred direction. By incorporating the training of Kriya Yoga into your every day lifestyles, you may embark on a transformative journey in the route of the final union with the Divine - Samadhi. May this e-book function a beacon of mild, predominant you inside the path of the belief of your actual Self and the ecstatic bliss of Samadhi.

Chapter 3: The Role Of Guru In Kriya Yoga

Understanding the Importance of a Guru

In the route of self-awareness, it's far often said that finding a actual guru is one of the most large milestones. A guru, in the context of Kriya Yoga, isn't best a teacher or a manual, but a non secular grasp who has attained enlightenment and possesses the expertise and belief to guide seekers within the route in their own self-consciousness. Understanding the importance of a guru is vital for each seeker on the route of Kriya Yoga.

A guru serves as a dwelling example of the divine potential inner every man or woman. They have traversed the direction themselves, experiencing the transformative strength of Kriya Yoga firsthand. Their presence and teachings inspire and ignite the inner flame of aspiration within the seeker, presenting a roadmap for the journey toward self-recognition.

One of the primary motives a guru is critical is their capability to transmit religious power or shaktipat. This divine energy, obtained through the guru's grace, awakens dormant spiritual schools within the seeker. This transmission isn't always in reality a switch of statistics but a profound energetic connection that quickens the seeker's development at the path.

Moreover, a guru possesses the capability to dispel doubts, make clear misconceptions, and answer questions that rise up on the religious journey. Through their steering, seekers can benefit a deeper know-how of the esoteric teachings of Kriya Yoga and navigate the intricacies of the course with clarity and self warranty.

A guru additionally performs the function of a compassionate pal, presenting aid and encouragement at some point of moments of doubt or religious stagnation. They offer solace and reassurance at some point of the difficult levels of the adventure, reminding seekers to live devoted and persevere in their exercising.

However, it's miles critical to method the guru-disciple dating with sincerity, humility, and discernment. Seekers want to cautiously select out a guru who resonates with their innermost being and aligns with the classes of Kriya Yoga. Once the guru is selected, it's miles crucial to give up to their guidance wholeheartedly, trusting in their facts and steerage.

In quit, facts the importance of a guru in the exercise of Kriya Yoga is critical for each seeker. A guru serves as a beacon of moderate, guiding seekers within the course of self-attention. They transmit religious energy, dispel doubts, and provide precious assist on the path. By selecting a guru with discernment and surrendering to their steering, seekers can accelerate their spiritual evolution and embark on a transformative journey in the direction of self-focus.

Finding a Genuine Guru for Kriya Yoga

Kriya Yoga is a profound spiritual workout that holds the capability to guide each seeker within the direction of self-interest. However, embarking on this transformative adventure calls for steering from a actual guru who possesses deep expertise and revel in in this historic artwork. In this subchapter, we're able to explore the developments to search for even as searching for a true guru for Kriya Yoga.

First and primary, a actual guru need to have a strong lineage and connection to the Kriya Yoga life-style. They need to be capable of hint their teachings once more to the remarkable masters who have illuminated this route through the some time. This ensures that the instructions they create are actual and rooted in the awareness passed down thru generations.

Additionally, a real guru need to own a deep information of the thoughts and practices of Kriya Yoga. They need to be well-versed within the philosophical foundations of this non secular course and be able to manual college students thru the severa levels of workout. A proper guru will not best provide theoretical know-how but may even offer realistic strategies and wearing events that assist human beings experience the transformative energy of Kriya Yoga.

Furthermore, a actual guru have to encompass the functions of compassion, humility, and unconditional love. They ought to be devoted to the welfare in their college college students and sincerely care approximately their non secular boom. A true guru will create a supportive and nurturing surroundings wherein seekers can freely particular their doubts and fears with out judgment. Their steering can be moderate, but business enterprise, helping university university college students triumph over limitations and progress on their spiritual journey.

It is likewise crucial to trying to find a guru who encourages impartial wondering and self-inquiry. A right guru will not impose their ideals or dogmas on their college college

college students however alternatively inspire them to find out and discover their very own truth. They will inspire seekers to impeach, inspect, and validate the instructions for themselves, fostering a revel in of self-empowerment and internal discernment.

Lastly, a proper guru will constantly emphasize the importance of ordinary exercising and willpower. They will manual university university college students in establishing a steady habitual, incorporating meditation, pranayama, and one-of-a-kind Kriya Yoga strategies into their each day lives. They will emphasize the want for staying power, perseverance, and backbone at the direction, information that self-cognizance is a slow method that requires steady strive.

In cease, finding a actual guru for Kriya Yoga is important for all of us embarking in this transformative adventure. By searching for a guru with a sturdy lineage, deep information, and embodying developments of compassion and humility, people can find out the guidance and help they want to navigate the course of Kriya Yoga correctly. Remember, the right guru will now not best mild up the manner but additionally empower seekers to recognize their private divinity.

Establishing a Guru-Disciple Relationship

In the vicinity of spiritual growth and self-reputation, the significance of a Guru-Disciple relationship can not be overstated. In the ancient workout of Kriya Yoga, this bond is considered critical for the seeker's journey towards self-recognition. Whether you're new to Kriya Yoga or were practising for a while, information and putting in place a Guru-Disciple dating is important for deepening your spiritual route.

The time period "Guru" actually interprets to "dispeller of darkness" in Sanskrit. A Guru is not handiest a trainer but a guide, mentor, and embodiment of attention. They possess the statistics and revel in vital to navigate the complexities of religious increase and enlightenment. A proper Guru holds the electricity to awaken the divine spark within the seeker, maximum essential them in the direction of self-awareness and liberation.

To installation a Guru-Disciple relationship, one need to method the hunt with sincerity, humility, and an open coronary coronary coronary heart. It is vital to analyze and discover a Guru who aligns in conjunction with your non secular aspirations and resonates with your innermost being. Once you have got got diagnosed a capability Guru, it is in truth beneficial to meet them in man or woman or via virtual manner to evaluate the compatibility of your energies.

A Guru-Disciple courting is built on a basis of remember, surrender, and devotion. The disciple need to give up their ego, doubts, and preconceived notions, permitting the Guru to guide them on their spiritual adventure. In return, the Guru gives spiritual teachings, practices, and steerage tailor-made to the disciple's particular wishes. This dating isn't always transactional but alternatively a sacred bond that transcends time and region.

Regular communique and interaction with the Guru are vital for the disciple's boom. The Guru imparts expertise and information via personal guidance, satsangs (spiritual gatherings), and initiation into better practices. The disciple ought to approach the ones interactions with a receptive mind, absorbing the training and enforcing them in their day by day life.

It is important to be aware that a Guru-Disciple courting isn't always constrained to bodily proximity. In today's digital age, seekers can connect to Gurus from precise factors of the sector thru on-line systems. The non secular strength and steering can be transmitted at some point of distances, permitting the seeker to revel in the Guru's records and beauty.

In end, putting in location a Guru-Disciple dating is a transformative step in the route of Kriya Yoga. It gives the seeker with the vital guidance, aid, and idea to improvement on their spiritual adventure. By surrendering to the Guru and cultivating a deep experience of devotion, the disciple opens themselves as a exquisite deal because the transformative power of self-interest and the final goal of Kriya Yoga – union with the divine.

The Guru's Role in Guiding the Seeker's Journey

In the profound religious direction of Kriya Yoga, the position of the guru is of paramount importance. The seeker embarks on a journey closer to self-popularity, and the guru acts as a guiding slight, illuminating the path and crucial the manner. The guru's position isn't always restricted to imparting information but extends to presenting help, notion, and steering in the course of the seeker's transformational journey.

One of the primary responsibilities of the guru is to transmit the teachings and techniques of Kriya Yoga to the seeker. These teachings are ancient and sacred, exceeded down through generations of enlightened masters. The guru imparts those teachings with utmost care and precision, making sure that the seeker receives the information in its purest form. Through this transmission, the seeker income access to powerful non secular device that may accelerate their development in the direction of self-consciousness.

However, the guru's characteristic is going beyond mere coaching. They characteristic a dwelling embodiment of the instructions, demonstrating the ideas of Kriya Yoga thru their very personal existence and movements. The guru's presence radiates information, compassion, and unconditional love, developing an surroundings conducive to spiritual increase. By observing the guru, the seeker learns no longer best from their terms however additionally from their manner of being.

The guru additionally plays a critical role in providing steerage and useful useful resource to the seeker in the course of their adventure.

As the seeker encounters challenges, doubts, and boundaries, the guru is there to offer solace, clarity, and encouragement. The guru's profound knowledge and enjoy help the seeker navigate through the complexities of the spiritual route, ensuring they live on route and avoid pitfalls.

Furthermore, the guru serves as a supply of idea for the seeker. By witnessing the guru's very very very own religious evolution and enlightenment, the seeker is stimulated to persevere in their exercising and attempt for self-interest. The guru's presence serves as a constant reminder of the final purpose and the limitless opportunities that lie earlier.

It is essential to phrase that locating the right guru is a deeply personal and intuitive system. The seeker need to pay attention to their inner voice and keep in thoughts their instincts whilst deciding on a guru. The guru-seeker courting is constructed on mutual keep in mind, appreciate, and devotion. When this bond is set up, the seeker can wholeheartedly surrender to the guru's steerage, facts that they may be in stable hands.

In give up, the guru's feature in guiding the seeker's adventure of self-awareness in Kriya Yoga is crucial. They aren't best instructors but additionally mentors, guides, and inspirations. With their interest, compassion, and useful useful resource, the guru empowers the seeker to go beyond obstacles, awaken their true capacity, and embark on a transformative non secular journey.

Chapter 4: The Science Of Kundalini Awakening

Introduction to Kundalini Energy

Kundalini energy, moreover known as the existence pressure or the divine energy, is a effective and transformative strain that is living inner each and each one of us. It is frequently defined as a coiled serpent, dormant at the lowest of the spine, organized to be woke up. In the ancient exercising of Kriya Yoga, the awakening of this Kundalini strength is considered vital for self-cognizance and spiritual growth.

This subchapter pastimes to provide an introduction to Kundalini strength, explaining its importance and the function it plays within the practice of Kriya Yoga. Whether you're a seasoned practitioner or a newcomer to the region of yoga and spirituality, understanding Kundalini electricity is critical for unlocking your complete potential and embarking on a profound adventure toward self-popularity.

Kundalini electricity is stated to be the supply of our power, creativity, and religious awakening. When awakened, it moves via the subtle energy channels referred to as nadis, purifying and energizing every thing of our being. This effective strength can result in profound recovery, heightened interest, and a deep enjoy of reference to the divine.

In this subchapter, we are able to delve into the numerous additives of Kundalini strength, exploring its basis, nature, and the manner of awakening. We will speak the chakras, the energy facilities along the backbone through which Kundalini power ascends, and the significance of balancing and harmonizing those centers.

Furthermore, we're capable of find out the practices and techniques that could facilitate the awakening and stable ascent of Kundalini strength. From pranayama (breathing physical activities) to asanas (yoga postures), mantra chanting, and meditation, each practice plays a vital role in getting geared up the frame, mind, and spirit for the effective awakening of Kundalini strength.

Throughout this subchapter, we also can deal with commonplace questions and worries that stand up whilst operating with Kundalini electricity, emphasizing the significance of guidance from an skilled trainer or guru. Kundalini awakening is a profound and doubtlessly severe enjoy, and right steering ensures a stable and transformative adventure.

Whether you're searching for self-cognizance, non secular boom, or definitely a deeper facts of the yogic direction, this subchapter will offer you with a stable basis to find out the place of Kundalini electricity. By harnessing this transformative pressure interior, you could liberate your most potential, wake up your divine nature, and embark on a profound journey within the path of self-focus thru the practice of Kriya Yoga.

Understanding the Chakras and their Significance

The historical workout of Kriya Yoga is a adventure towards self-interest, guiding seekers on a course of religious increase and enlightenment. At the center of this profound exercise lies the know-how and activation of the chakras – energy facilities that exist within the diffused frame.

The chakras are frequently defined as spinning wheels of power positioned alongside the backbone, every corresponding to important components of our physical, emotional, and non secular properly-being. There are seven maximum crucial chakras, starting from the lowest of the backbone and growing to the crown of the top.

The first chakra, known as the Muladhara or the Root Chakra, is related to our basis, balance, and feel of belonging. It is represented thru the colour crimson and governs our physical fitness, survival instincts, and connection to the material international.

Moving upwards, the second one chakra, called Svadhisthana or the Sacral Chakra, is associated with creativity, ardour, and sexuality. It is represented thru the colour orange and influences our capability to revel in delight, connect with others emotionally, and embody our sensuality.

The 1/three chakra, Manipura or the Solar Plexus Chakra, is positioned inside the place of the navel and is associated with private electricity, arrogance, and confidence. Represented with the aid of the color yellow, it governs our self-control, motivation, and capability to achieve this.

The fourth chakra, Anahata or the Heart Chakra, is placed within the middle of the chest and is related to love, compassion, and emotional restoration. Represented via way of the shade green, it connects us to the strength of unconditional love, allowing us to provide and acquire love freely.

Moving in addition up, the fifth chakra, Vishuddha or the Throat Chakra, is related to conversation, self-expression, and authenticity. Represented with the resource of the coloration blue, it governs our functionality to talk our truth, pay hobby attentively, and particular ourselves creatively.

The sixth chakra, Ajna or the Third Eye Chakra, is positioned a number of the eyebrows and is related to intuition, understanding, and inner vision. Represented with the resource of the colour indigo, it lets in us to get proper of entry to our higher reputation, enhance our instinct, and advantage clarity of concept.

Finally, the 7th chakra, Sahasrara or the Crown Chakra, is placed at the pinnacle of the pinnacle and represents our connection to the divine. Represented by way of the coloration violet or white, it's far associated with spiritual awakening, enlightenment, and the combination of our better self.

Understanding the importance of the chakras is essential for practitioners of Kriya Yoga as it allows them to harmonize and balance those energy facilities, as a result selling holistic well-being. Through numerous Kriya Yoga techniques which includes pranayama (respiratory carrying activities), meditation, and asanas (yoga postures), you may simply spark off and purify the chakras, permitting the free go with the flow of energy in a few unspecified time within the destiny of the frame.

By walking with the chakras, humans can cope with imbalances, heal emotional wounds, and cultivate a deeper connection with their higher self. This information of the chakras and their significance now not quality complements our bodily and emotional health but moreover opens the door to religious growth, self-attention, and a profound enjoy of inner peace.

Whether you're new to Kriya Yoga or already on the course, delving into the profound statistics of the chakras and their importance will definitely deepen your workout and guide you in the course of self-recognition – a adventure nicely really well worth challenge for seekers from all walks of life.

Techniques for Safely Awakening the Kundalini

The awakening of the Kundalini power, frequently known as the dormant religious power interior each person, is a profound and transformative enjoy. However, it's miles vital to approach this approach with caution and information to make certain a strong and harmonious awakening. In this subchapter, we are able to explore a few techniques for efficaciously awakening the Kundalini, specifically designed for practitioners of Kriya Yoga.

1. Preparation and Alignment: Before attempting any Kundalini awakening strategies, it is vital to put together the body and mind. Regular exercising of asanas (yoga postures) and pranayama (breathing physical video games) allows to purify and decorate the bodily frame, even as meditation and mantra chanting create a snug and focused

mind. This alignment of body and mind creates a solid basis for Kundalini awakening.

2. Guidance from a Qualified Teacher: Kundalini awakening is a profound adventure, and having a licensed trainer or guru to manual you through the approach is beneficial. A teacher can offer personalized guidance, display your improvement, and offer manual sooner or later of any worrying situations which could upward push up.

3. Gradual Awakening: It is critical to awaken the Kundalini little by little, permitting the power to go with the float manifestly via the only of a kind energy facilities (chakras) along the spine. Starting with mild practices like spinal respiration and power recognition bodily games, progressively development closer to extra superior techniques together with Kriya Yoga.

4. Balancing the Energy: Kundalini awakening can generate extreme power, and it's far important to stability and harmonize this strength at a few degree inside the body. This

may be finished via normal exercise of Kriya Yoga strategies, which comprise specific breath control, power locks, and meditation practices. These techniques help to channel the Kundalini strength upwards, purifying and balancing the chakras alongside the way.

five. Self-Awareness and Listening to the Body: Throughout the Kundalini awakening procedure, it's far critical to domesticate self-popularity and concentrate to the body's alerts. If any pain or imbalance arises, it's miles critical to regulate the workout consequently or are searching for guidance from a licensed trainer.

Remember, Kundalini awakening is a deeply private and transformative journey. The strategies stated here are truely the top of the iceberg. It is important to approach this approach with humility, staying power, and appreciate for the electricity of the Kundalini electricity. With right steerage, willpower, and normal practice of Kriya Yoga, each person can correctly embark on the route of

Kundalini awakening and enjoy the profound self-cognizance it offers.

Harnessing the Power of Kundalini for Self-Realization

Kriya Yoga: A Journey Towards Self-Realization for Every Seeker

Introduction:

In the location of non secular practices, Kriya Yoga stands proud as a profound and transformative course within the direction of self-popularity. At the coronary coronary heart of this ancient exercising lies the awakening and harnessing of the Kundalini electricity, a dormant stress that is living interior each person. This subchapter explores the importance of Kundalini in the adventure within the course of self-reputation and how Kriya Yoga offers a systematic method to free up its exceptional power.

Understanding Kundalini Energy:

Kundalini, often referred to as the "serpent strength," represents the dormant non secular power lying coiled at the base of the spine. This effective pressure, at the identical time as awoke, has the capacity to raise recognition, deepen religious reviews, and bring about profound inner transformation. It is the important thing to unlocking the significant reservoir of untapped power indoors us.

The Power of Self-Realization:

Self-focus is the final goal of Kriya Yoga – the belief of our actual nature and the cohesion of the person self with the cosmic consciousness. By harnessing the strength of Kundalini, practitioners embark on a adventure of self-discovery, transcending barriers, and experiencing a deeper reference to the divine.

Kriya Yoga: The Path to Awakening Kundalini:

Kriya Yoga gives a scientific and scientific method to evoke and channel the dormant

Kundalini power. Through a mixture of particular breathing techniques, bodily postures, mantra recitation, and meditation, practitioners discover ways to awaken and direct the glide of Kundalini power alongside the backbone, regularly ascending inside the route of higher states of attention.

Benefits of Harnessing Kundalini Energy:

As practitioners development at the route of Kriya Yoga, they start to experience a large number of advantages. These consist of progressed bodily electricity, intellectual readability, emotional stability, more potent creativity, heightened instinct, and a deep feel of inner peace. The woke up Kundalini electricity purifies the body and thoughts, facilitating the elimination of blockages and negativities, leading to holistic nicely-being.

Precautions and Guidance:

It is crucial to approach the awakening of Kundalini with proper steerage and caution. In the subchapter, the e-book emphasizes the significance of seeking out steerage from an skilled instructor and jogging within the path of beneath their supervision. Kundalini awakening may be intense and overwhelming, and a pro instructor can provide the crucial guide and guidance to navigate via the way efficaciously.

Chapter 5: Navigating Obstacles At The Kriya Yoga Path

Dealing with Physical and Mental Challenges

In the adventure in the route of self-attention, it is vital to address each physical and highbrow worrying situations that one may additionally moreover come upon along the way. Kriya Yoga, a transformative exercise rooted in historic teachings, offers precious tools to assist human beings correctly address the ones obstacles.

Physical disturbing conditions can show up in numerous bureaucracy, which include continual contamination, physical disabilities, or even quick illnesses. Kriya Yoga emphasizes the significance of preserving a healthy frame to manual the spiritual adventure. By running closer to specific asanas (postures) and pranayama (breathing techniques), humans can domesticate physical strength and flexibility, on the equal time as also improving normal well-being. Regular exercise of Kriya Yoga permits the body to growth resilience, allowing practitioners to triumph over bodily traumatic situations with greater ease.

Mental demanding conditions, however, can show up as pressure, tension, melancholy, or loss of readability. Kriya Yoga offers powerful strategies to calm and awareness the thoughts. Through meditation and attention bodily video games, practitioners can enlarge highbrow clarity, emotional stability, and a deeper information of themselves. These practices assist people to effectively manipulate their mind and emotions, letting them navigate thru highbrow stressful situations with more resilience.

Kriya Yoga additionally recognizes the interconnectedness of the mind and frame. It teaches that bodily and intellectual well-being are deeply intertwined, and an imbalance in you can have an effect on the opposite. By addressing each additives concurrently, Kriya Yoga gives a holistic technique to handling stressful situations.

Furthermore, Kriya Yoga teaches human beings to growth a excellent attitude and cultivate gratitude, even in the face of adversity. This attitude shift lets in practitioners to view worrying situations as possibilities for growth and self-discovery. By embracing traumatic conditions as a part of the adventure, individuals can redesign limitations into stepping stones toward self-focus.

In conclusion, Kriya Yoga offers valuable steerage for anybody, which includes folks that are in particular inquisitive about the workout of Kriya Yoga. By incorporating bodily asanas, pranayama, meditation, and awareness wearing sports, human beings can efficiently deal with both bodily and intellectual traumatic conditions. This holistic technique fosters resilience, clarity, and a terrific mindset, permitting people to navigate the adventure closer to self-reputation with grace and electricity. Whether you're a amateur or an skilled seeker, the instructions of Kriya Yoga may be a transformative device to help you triumph over boundaries and embrace the course in the direction of self-interest.

Overcoming Doubts and Inner Resistance

Overcoming Doubts and Inner Resistance

Introduction:

In the pursuit of self-consciousness, doubts and internal resistance frequently end up ambitious obstacles on the direction of spiritual increase. Many seekers of fact, together with the ones education Kriya Yoga, stumble upon moments of uncertainty and resistance that can prevent their improvement. However, it's miles essential to well known that the ones doubts and inner resistance are herbal and may be conquer with the right approach and mind-set.

Understanding Doubts:

Doubts get up from the intellect's try and apprehend the divine mysteries past its restricted scope. They may additionally

70

moreover stem from societal conditioning, fear of the unknown, or the ego's reluctance to surrender manipulate. It is crucial to understand that doubts aren't inherently lousy; they might function catalysts for deeper inquiry and facts. By embracing doubts as possibilities for non secular boom, seekers can redesign them into stepping stones within the direction of self-recognition.

Overcoming Inner Resistance:

Inner resistance, often manifested as a sense of fear or reluctance, can stand up even as human beings are confronted with the profound modifications introduced about thru non secular practices like Kriya Yoga. This resistance can stem from attachment to vintage patterns, the concern of dropping one's identification, or the pain related to stepping outside one's consolation area. It is essential to widely known that inner resistance is a natural safety mechanism of the ego, striving to maintain the popularity quo.

Strategies for Overcoming Doubts and Inner Resistance:

1. Cultivate Self-Awareness: Developing a deep statistics of oneself, collectively with one's fears, insecurities, and restricting beliefs, is vital. Self-cognizance permits seekers to understand doubts and internal resistance when they upward thrust up and address them consciously.

2. Seek Guidance: Connecting with skilled teachers and like-minded humans who've traversed comparable paths can offer valuable assist and steerage. Their information and insights can assist alleviate doubts and encourage perseverance inside the face of internal resistance.

three. Surrender to the Process: By surrendering to the higher electricity or divine intelligence, seekers can relinquish manipulate and maintain in thoughts inside the transformative adventure of self-reputation. Surrendering permits one to allow flow of doubts and resistance, paving the way for profound non secular reviews.

four. Practice Patience and Persistence: The course in the direction of self-focus is usually a lengthy and onerous one. Patience and endurance are essential virtues as doubts and resistance can also resurface at one in all a kind stages of the adventure. Trust within the way and remain devoted to the workout of Kriya Yoga.

Addressing Spiritual Plateaus and Lack of Progress

In the journey of self-recognition, seekers frequently encounter religious plateaus and periods of stagnation. These stages may be disheartening and might lead one to question their willpower to the direction of self-discovery. However, it's miles critical to recognize that these plateaus are a natural part of the religious journey, and that they provide precious opportunities for boom and transformation.

Kriya Yoga, a profound historical exercise, gives powerful equipment to overcome those plateaus and reignite the spark of improvement. It offers a complete approach to spirituality, encompassing physical, intellectual, and non secular elements, making it reachable to absolutely everyone, regardless of their ancient past or ideals.

One of the principle motives for encountering a religious plateau is the lack of information and information of the diffused dynamics of the exercising. Kriya Yoga emphasizes the significance of self-test and self-mirrored photo. By deepening our records of our personal mind, emotions, and idea styles, we're able to pick out the limitations that limit our development and cope with them correctly.

Another commonplace cause of religious stagnation is a loss of area and consistency in our exercise. Kriya Yoga encourages seekers to set up a regular recurring, which consist of meditation, pranayama (breathing physical video games), and asanas (bodily postures). By dedicating time and effort to the ones practices, we create a fertile ground for spiritual boom and transcendence.

Additionally, it's far important to cultivate staying power and perseverance on the non secular direction. Progress might not continually be linear; it regularly takes vicinity in cycles, with intervals of rapid development observed through plateaus. Understanding that those plateaus are transient and a part of the herbal rhythm of religious evolution can help us hold our motivation and determination.

Kriya Yoga additionally emphasizes the significance of searching for steerage from professional teachers or mentors. These human beings can offer valuable insights and useful resource, supporting us navigate through the worrying situations and plateaus with readability and know-how.

Lastly, it is essential to cultivate a enjoy of give up and acquire as right with within the

Divine. By relinquishing our attachment to unique outcomes or expectations, we create place for the universe to guide and uplift us. This surrender permits us to permit pass of the ego's desire for improvement and as a substitute hobby on the winning second, embracing the adventure itself because the final cause.

In stop, spiritual plateaus and shortage of development are common studies at the course of self-attention. Through the exercise of Kriya Yoga, you can nevertheless overcome those traumatic conditions and keep their adventure towards self-discovery. By developing self-interest, area, staying strength, searching for guidance, and cultivating give up, we will pass beyond the ones plateaus and enjoy profound boom and transformation on our non secular path. Kriya Yoga is a effective device that might help each seeker in carrying out their maximum capability and assignment self-recognition.

Cultivating Patience and Persistence in Practice

Cultivating Patience and Persistence in Practice

In the course of Kriya Yoga, staying power and staying energy are two essential tendencies that every seeker ought to try and cultivate. These virtues no longer handiest make certain development in our religious journey however also help us navigate the demanding situations and barriers that can upward push up alongside the way. Patience and staying electricity are just like the dual pillars that assist our exercising, permitting us to enlarge a deep reference to our internal self and obtain self-attention.

Patience is a fantastic feature that allows us to stay calm and composed, even within the face of troubles and setbacks. In the arena of Kriya Yoga, patience is needed as we embark at the path of self-discovery. It reminds us that the adventure within the path of self-cognizance is not a quick restore but a slow manner that calls for time, electricity of mind, and try. By cultivating staying energy, we discover ways to apprehend the prevailing 2nd and recollect in the divine timing of our non secular boom. We understand that actual transformation can't be rushed but unfolds genuinely even as we're organized to get hold of it.

Persistence is some other essential superb that propels us in advance on the route of Kriya Yoga. It is the unwavering determination to our exercising, although the consequences might not be immediately obvious. Through staying energy, we increase the electricity to overcome boundaries and withstand the enticements to wasteland our religious route. It is thru chronic workout that we harness the power of Kriya Yoga and revel in its profound consequences on our thoughts, body, and soul. Like a normal flame, staying power continues our non secular hearth alive, guiding us in the route of self-reputation.

In the pursuit of endurance and staying power, we ought to recollect that each seeker's adventure is precise. Each man or woman progresses at their non-public pace, and comparing ourselves to others best hinders our growth. Kriya Yoga teaches us to hobby on our personal exercising, embracing the method in place of fixating at the outcome. By cultivating persistence and endurance, we create a fertile ground for self-recognition to blossom.

In stop, the subchapter "Cultivating Patience and Persistence in Practice" emphasizes the significance of those virtues within the exercising of Kriya Yoga. Patience allows us to give up to the divine timing of our non secular increase, while endurance keeps us dedicated to our exercise, even in the face of annoying conditions. Through the ones trends, we expand a deeper reference to our inner self and pave the manner for self-attention. Remember, the journey of Kriya Yoga isn't a sprint however a marathon, and it is thru staying power and staying electricity that we will sincerely redesign ourselves and experience the profound blessings of this sacred route.

Chapter 6: Integrating Kriya Yoga Into Daily Life

Applying Kriya Yoga Principles to Relationships

In our journey toward self-interest, it is crucial to apprehend that our relationships play a crucial role in our spiritual growth. Kriya Yoga, a direction of self-discovery and transformation, offers profound requirements which can assist us domesticate harmonious and welcoming connections with others.

One of the essential teachings of Kriya Yoga is the concept of oneness – the knowledge that we're all interconnected and a part of a divine complete. This principle can revolutionize the manner we technique our relationships. When we apprehend the divinity internal ourselves and others, we obviously increase compassion, respect, and kindness within the course of all and sundry we encounter.

Another key precept of Kriya Yoga is the cultivation of internal stillness and quietness through meditation. By often running in the direction of meditation, we expand a more capability to live focused and found in our relationships. This permits us to concentrate more attentively, reply with clarity and know-how, and preserve a enjoy of inner peace even in tough conditions. Through meditation, we can also get right of entry to our intuition, which permits us make choices that are aligned with our better reason and make contributions undoubtedly to our relationships.

Kriya Yoga emphasizes the significance of self-control and self-awareness. Applying these thoughts to relationships way taking duty for our very very very own emotions, mind, and movements. By training energy of mind, we learn how to reply in area of react swiftly, fostering extra healthful and extra harmonious interactions. Self-focus allows us pick out our personal styles and triggers, permitting us to behave from an area of conscious preference and keep away from unnecessary conflicts and misunderstandings.

Additionally, Kriya Yoga teaches the electricity of love and forgiveness. Love is the using stress at the back of all relationships, and at the same time as we technique others with love and recognition, we create an surroundings of trust and information. Forgiveness, both in the direction of ourselves and others, is vital for freeing emotional baggage and cultivating a revel in of freedom and liberation inner our relationships.

By using Kriya Yoga principles to our relationships, we're capable of remodel them proper right into a sacred vicinity for increase, recovery, and mutual evolution. Whether it is with our family, friends, or partners, each interplay will become an possibility to deepen our religious understanding, expand our capability for love and compassion, and in the end, apprehend our actual nature.

Regardless of your background or beliefs, Kriya Yoga offers worthwhile insights and practices that may decorate your relationships and bring greater achievement and joy into your lifestyles. Embrace those ideas, embark for your journey within the course of self-interest, and watch as your relationships blossom into profound connections of love and concord.

Balancing Work, Family, and Spiritual Practice

In our fast-paced and stressful global, finding stability among work, circle of relatives, and spiritual exercise can frequently look like an not possible mission. The pressures of each day lifestyles, the obligations we inventory, and the regular desires on our time can leave us feeling crushed and disconnected from our spiritual selves. However, for people who are on the course of Kriya Yoga, it's miles essential to find this stability if you want to domesticate internal peace, self-attention, and a harmonious life.

Work, circle of relatives, and non secular workout are three essential factors of our lives that need to not be treated as separate entities, however rather as interconnected elements that assist and nourish each different. While it is able to appear hard, integrating the ones three additives can deliver profound achievement and a experience of purpose to our lives.

First and primary, it's miles critical to apprehend that our spiritual exercise need to no longer be limited to a particular time or vicinity. It need to permeate every component of our lives, together with our paintings and own family lifestyles. By infusing our every day obligations and interactions with mindfulness, compassion, and gratitude, we're able to rework ordinary moments into sacred ones.

One way to gain this integration is with the aid of using placing smooth priorities and barriers. It is important to allocate dedicated time for each of those elements, making sure that none is omitted. By efficaciously managing our time and strength, we create location for self-care, family bonding, and non secular growth. This also can require making aware selections, collectively with decreasing non-crucial commitments or delegating obligations each time possible.

Additionally, it's far important to talk brazenly and sincerely with our cherished ones approximately the significance of our religious practice. By concerning them in our journey and seeking out their assist, we are able to foster a supportive environment that nurtures our increase and encourages their very private religious exploration.

Furthermore, working towards energy of will and self-care is important in keeping this stability. Regularly challenge sports that refill and rejuvenate us, which include meditation, yoga, or nature walks, ensures that we are mentally, emotionally, and bodily prepared to satisfy our responsibilities and interact in reality with our loved ones.

Ultimately, locating stability among art work, family, and religious exercise is a non-forestall approach of self-discovery and model. It requires a deep willpower to our non secular course and a willingness to prioritize our well-being and private boom. By integrating those factors, we're able to lead enjoyable lives, radiate positivity, and inspire others to embark on their personal adventure of self-cognizance thru Kriya Yoga.

Creating a Sacred Space for Regular Sadhana

In the course of Kriya Yoga, regular sadhana, or spiritual workout, is of immoderate significance. It is through ordinary and committed exercising that we're capable to hook up with our real selves and realise our most functionality. However, if you need to domesticate a deep and big exercise, it's far critical to create a sacred area that enables and nourishes our non secular journey.

A sacred area is not restrained to a bodily area; it's far a state of thoughts, an internal sanctuary where we can dive deep into our exercise with out distractions. Whether you've got were given a dedicated room or a small nook in your property, the key's to infuse it with remarkable strength and purpose. Here are a few steps that will help you create a sacred vicinity in your ordinary sadhana:

1. Choose a region: Find a quiet and secluded place in your private home wherein you can workout undisturbed. It is probably a spare room, a corner of your bedroom, or perhaps an opening for your garden. Ensure that the space is clean, well-ventilated, and unfastened from muddle.

2. Clear the electricity: Before you start putting in place your sacred space, cleanse the region energetically. Burn some sage or incense, sprinkle holy water, or use any purification ritual that resonates with you. This will help dispose of any awful energy and create a sparkling and alluring ecosystem.

3. Decorate mindfully: Personalize your sacred place with gadgets and logos that inspire and uplift you. This need to embody statues or snap shots of religious masters, candles, vegetation, crystals, or sacred texts. Choose gadgets that have a deep which

means for you and evoke a revel in of reverence.

four. Establish a focus: Set up a focus on your sacred area to direct your attention inside the direction of exercising. This may be a small altar with a candle or a image of your preferred deity. Having a focal point allows to middle and pay interest the mind, bearing in mind a deeper meditation experience.

5. Create a peaceful atmosphere: Enhance the surroundings of your sacred space through playing smooth instrumental track or chanting mantras in the background. Consider the usage of important oils or incense to infuse the air with a chilled perfume. The cause is to create an environment that promotes tranquility and rest.

Remember, the sacred region you create is a reflection of your inner state. It is a sanctuary wherein you can allow pass of the outside global and dive deep into the nation-states of your very non-public being. Regularly spending time on this vicinity will now not best deepen your sadhana but moreover deliver a feel of peace and concord to your ordinary life.

So, take some time to create a sacred place that resonates along with your soul and permits your non secular journey. Embrace the splendor of Kriya Yoga and allow your sacred location emerge as a gateway to self-popularity for every seeker.

Living a Mindful and Conscious Life

In present day day rapid-paced international, it is easy to get stuck up in the each day grind and lose sight of what without a doubt topics. We often find ourselves dashing from one task to every extraordinary, without taking the time to pause and replicate on our movements. However, via incorporating mindfulness and reputation into our lives, we are able to experience a profound transformation that effects in self-popularity and inner peace. This subchapter titled "Living a Mindful and Conscious Life" delves into the essence of Kriya Yoga and how it can manual us closer to a extra pleasing existence.

Kriya Yoga, a non secular exercising rooted in historic information, offers a powerful technique for self-interest. It invitations anyone, no matter their historical past or beliefs, to embark on a adventure of self-discovery and internal increase. At its center, Kriya Yoga teaches us to stay each moment with reason and reputation. It emphasizes the importance of being absolutely present within the here and now, as opposed to dwelling on the beyond or demanding approximately the destiny.

To stay a aware lifestyles manner to cultivate a deep feel of awareness and interest inside the path of our mind, emotions, and moves. It calls for us to have a take a look at ourselves with out judgment, permitting us to gain perception into our patterns and conditioning. By jogging closer to mindfulness, we're capable of expand a more understanding of ourselves and the area spherical us, leading to a greater compassionate and empathetic lifestyles.

Consciousness, rather, refers back to the kingdom of being wide awake and aware about our innermost essence. It is the capability to go beyond the constraints of the ego and connect with our real nature. Through the workout of Kriya Yoga, we're able to awaken our popularity and faucet into the limitless properly of information and love this is residing internal us.

Living a aware and aware life involves incorporating severa practices into our day by day recurring. These can also encompass meditation, breathwork, self-reflected picture, and conscious motion. By sporting out those practices, we are able to cultivate a deep experience of internal peace, stability, and resilience.

In this subchapter, you can explore the simplest-of-a-type strategies and concepts of Kriya Yoga that allow you to include a conscious and conscious life. You will discover ways to integrate the ones practices into your each day habitual and discover the profound impact they may must your fashionable well-being.

Whether you are a seasoned practitioner of Kriya Yoga or new to this non secular course, this subchapter will offer you with precious insights and realistic equipment to live a more conscious and aware existence. By embracing those teachings, you could embark on a transformative adventure within the course of self-awareness and inner success.

Chapter 7: Advanced Practices In Kriya Yoga

Exploring Advanced Pranayama Techniques

In the historic workout of Kriya Yoga, the art work of breath control performs a important function in carrying out self-hobby. Pranayama, the technological understanding of regulating the breath, goes beyond mere respiration bodily video games to delve into the diffused power structures of the frame. In this subchapter, we are able to find out advanced pranayama techniques that can deepen your know-how of Kriya Yoga and beautify your religious adventure.

One of the advanced pranayama strategies is Nadi Shodhana, additionally known as change nostril respiration. This technique balances the left and proper electricity channels in the frame, promoting concord and readability of thoughts. By the use of the thumb and ring finger to govern the nostrils, you could adjust the glide of breath, bearing in mind the purification and rejuvenation of the nadis, or strength channels.

Another powerful approach is Kapalabhati, or cranium shining breath. This dynamic pranayama entails forceful exhalations and passive inhalations, stimulating the sun plexus and cleaning the respiratory device. Kapalabhati now not nice strengthens the belly muscular tissues but additionally energizes the mind, bringing approximately mental readability and heightened consciousness.

In the world of advanced pranayama, one encounters the exercising of Kumbhaka, or breath retention. This approach includes maintaining the breath after inhalation (Antar Kumbhaka) or after exhalation (Bahya Kumbhaka). Through managed breath retention, the practitioner critiques a deep stillness and growth of interest. Kumbhaka is a powerful device for cultivating attention and tapping into the massive reservoirs of energy inside.

Additionally, Bhramari Pranayama, or humming bee breath, is a complicated method that uses the energy of sound vibrations. By remaining the ears with the thumbs and making a low buzzing sound at the same time as exhaling, one must awaken the internal sound current and get right of get entry to to higher states of attention. Bhramari Pranayama is particularly useful for calming the mind, reducing tension, and selling a experience of inner peace.

It is critical to phrase that superior pranayama techniques want to be practiced beneath the steerage of an professional teacher. These practices require right information, vicinity, and slow improvement to make certain protection and effectiveness. Regular exercising of superior pranayama can cause profound non secular research, prolonged electricity, and a deeper reference to one's genuine Self.

In quit, exploring superior pranayama techniques in the context of Kriya Yoga opens up new dimensions of self-attention. By incorporating the ones practices into your non secular journey, you may launch the hidden capability interior and enjoy the transformative energy of the breath. May your exploration of advanced pranayama techniques deepen your know-how of Kriya Yoga and bring you toward the conclusion of your real nature.

Deepening Meditation through Advanced Methods

Deepening Meditation through Advanced Methods

Meditation is a effective practice that permits people to connect to their inner selves and enjoy a nation of profound peace and clarity. In the arena of Kriya Yoga, meditation takes on an entire new diploma of significance, imparting seekers a pathway towards self-cognizance and non secular enlightenment. Building upon the foundational techniques of Kriya Yoga, superior methods of deepening meditation can unfastened up even extra depths of attention and bliss.

One of the critical element elements of superior meditation in Kriya Yoga is the refinement of breath control. In this degree, practitioners are brought to pranayama, the historic yogic technology of breath. By consciously regulating the breath, you may honestly harness the existence strain strength and direct it in the route of the awakening of better states of cognizance. Advanced pranayama techniques, consisting of Nadi Shodhana (exchange nostril respiration) and Kumbhaka (breath retention), permit the seeker to purify the subtle power channels and awaken dormant spiritual schools.

Another essential factor of deepening meditation in Kriya Yoga is the exercising of mantra repetition. Mantras are sacred sounds or terms which have a vibrational impact at the mind and body. By repeating a particular mantra in a few unspecified time in the destiny of meditation, the seeker can deepen their awareness and go beyond the limitations of the regular mind. Advanced practitioners are initiated into the practice of japa meditation, in which they repeat their selected mantra with each breath, allowing the sound to permeate their entire being and dissolve the bounds of the ego.

Visualization strategies additionally play a vital feature in advanced meditation. Through the energy of creativeness, practitioners can create colourful intellectual pictures of divine office work or religious symbols. By that specialize in the ones visualizations at some stage in meditation, you could nevertheless access better geographical areas of attention and accumulate profound insights and steerage from the divine. Visualization strategies in Kriya Yoga assist to cultivate interest, expand recognition, and awaken the dormant powers of intuition and creativity.

As the seeker progresses in their adventure within the route of self-focus, they may moreover find out the practice of meditation on inner mild and sound. With steering from an expert instructor, the practitioner can turn their hobby inward and discover the nation-states of natural attention thru the belief of internal light and the diffused sound of Aum. These superior techniques allow the seeker to transcend the physical senses and revel in the countless and everlasting nature in their real self.

Deepening meditation through advanced strategies in Kriya Yoga requires dedication, field, and a sincere choice for self-consciousness. It is a transformative journey that takes the practitioner beyond the sector of the regular and into the arena of the brilliant. By incorporating the ones superior strategies into their meditation workout, seekers of all backgrounds and degrees of revel in can free up the door to self-reputation and embark on a lifelong journey closer to internal peace, achievement, and religious awakening.

Advancing Kundalini Awakening and Control

In the magical realm of non secular practices, Kundalini awakening holds a massive vicinity. It is a profound adventure towards self-popularity, offering a gateway to higher states of awareness. For seekers on the course of Kriya Yoga, understanding and harnessing the electricity of Kundalini is of excessive importance.

Kundalini, regularly symbolized as a coiled serpent at the lowest of the spine, represents the dormant religious power internal every person. Through committed exercising and proper steering, this power may be woke up and channeled to traverse the seven chakras, or electricity centers, inside the body. The end result is an progressed united states of attention and a deep connection with our authentic selves.

To boom on the path of Kundalini awakening, it's far critical to domesticate a strong foundation in Kriya Yoga. This ancient yogic technique combines breath manipulate, meditation, and bodily postures to harmonize the mind, frame, and spirit. By running in the route of Kriya Yoga diligently, you can purify the subtle strength channels within the body, permitting the Kundalini to rise without problems and efficiently.

However, Kundalini awakening isn't a journey to be taken gently. It requires staying power, region, and steerage from an professional trainer. The machine may be excessive, as dormant feelings and unresolved problems can also additionally floor in some unspecified time in the future of the awakening. Therefore, it's far vital to method this practice with reverence and admire, honoring the transformative energy it holds.

To strengthen in Kundalini manage, one need to learn how to balance the upward movement of strength with stability and grounding. This includes cultivating a sturdy bodily and intellectual basis thru everyday asana exercise, pranayama, and meditation. Developing a deep sense of self-reputation permits us to navigate the powerful power shifts that accompany Kundalini awakening.

Furthermore, integrating spiritual practices into our each day lives is crucial for keeping the improvement made in this direction. By incorporating mindfulness, powerful affirmations, and aware dwelling, we create a conducive environment for Kundalini to flourish. It is thru constant attempt and determination that we are able to hold to enhance at the direction of self-awareness.

In give up, advancing Kundalini awakening and manage is a profound adventure that requires energy of will and perseverance. By embracing the lessons and practices of Kriya Yoga, we are able to wake up the dormant Kundalini strength and experience profound transformation. However, it's miles essential to method this direction with warning, searching out steering from experienced teachers and cultivating a sturdy basis in bodily and spiritual practices. With honest attempt and a receptive mind, Kundalini can grow to be a powerful excellent friend on our adventure inside the course of self-interest, bringing us in the direction of our maximum capability.

The Role of Divine Love in Kriya Yoga

The Role of Divine Love in Kriya Yoga

Kriya Yoga, a profound spiritual course, offers a transformative adventure inside the direction of self-popularity for seekers from all walks of existence. At its middle, Kriya Yoga teaches the paintings of connecting with the divine internal us, and in doing so, it unveils the energy of divine love. This subchapter explores the pivotal function that divine love performs in Kriya Yoga and how it is able to certainly impact each individual, irrespective of their history or beliefs.

Divine love, regularly called unconditional love or natural love, is the essence of Kriya Yoga. It is the boundless love that emanates from the divine deliver, encompassing all beings and introduction itself. Through the exercise of Kriya Yoga, seekers learn how to faucet into this countless reservoir of love and permit it to permeate their complete being.

One of the principle features of Kriya Yoga is to dissolve the phantasm of separateness and domesticate a enjoy of cohesion with the divine and all life bureaucracy. Divine love serves because the bridge that connects us with this normal oneness. It is through love that we understand the divine presence in ourselves and others, fostering compassion, know-how, and beauty.

Kriya Yoga practitioners often experience a profound experience of internal peace, satisfaction, and fulfillment. This is due to the truth divine love, when accessed and allowed to waft freely, dissolves all fears, anxieties, and barriers that forestall our religious boom. It opens the doors to profound recovery, forgiveness, and the awakening of our real nature.

In Kriya Yoga, love isn't always absolutely a sentimental or emotional united states of america, but a transformative pressure that has the strength to purify the thoughts, frame, and soul. It is thru the cultivation of divine love that seekers can cross beyond the ego and its attachments, freeing themselves from the cycle of struggling and locating a deep enjoy of motive and achievement.

Regardless of one's spiritual or religious history, Kriya Yoga offers a everyday path that embraces the essence of divine love. It invitations everybody to discover and revel in the transformative electricity of love in their lives, fostering a experience of solidarity, concord, and peace inner themselves and the area spherical them.

In forestall, the placement of divine love in Kriya Yoga is important to the course of self-attention. It is thru the cultivation of divine love that seekers can enjoy profound recuperation, transcendence of boundaries, and a deep reference to the divine inside. By embracing love because the guiding stress in their lives, practitioners of Kriya Yoga can embark on a transformative adventure closer to self-awareness, locating actual motive, pleasure, and success along the way.

Chapter 8: The Journey To Self-Realization

Recognizing and Embracing the True Self

In the journey inside the path of self-reputation, one of the fundamental factors is recognizing and embracing the genuine self. This is a profound concept that lies on the coronary coronary heart of Kriya Yoga, a path that leads every seeker within the path of the notion in their inner divinity. Whether you're a devoted practitioner of Kriya Yoga or truly curious about exploring the depths of your being, knowledge and embracing your real self is a transformative and enlightening gadget.

The actual self, often known as the soul or the better self, is the essence of who we truely are beyond our physical our bodies and fleeting identities. It is the eternal and unchanging problem of our being that is related to the divine supply. Recognizing this truth permits us to tap into our limitless capability and revel in a profound revel in of fulfillment and motive in our lives.

Kriya Yoga presents practical equipment and strategies to help us apprehend and embody our real self. Through the workout of asanas (physical postures), pranayama (breath manage), and meditation, we are able to step by step peel away the layers of conditioning and societal expectancies that have veiled our real nature. As we delve deeper into our exercise, we start to revel in moments of clarity and glimpses of our real self shining through.

Embracing the proper self goes past highbrow know-how; it's far an experiential adventure that calls for self-meditated image, self-reputation, and self-love. It calls for us to allow circulate of our ego-pushed goals and attachments and surrender to the go with the flow of existence. By embracing our actual self, we align ourselves with the divine will and revel in a feel of crew spirit with all creation.

Recognizing and embracing the right self isn't restrained to the context of Kriya Yoga; it's miles a popular idea that holds relevance for everybody. In a international whole of distractions and outside affects, it is straightforward to lose contact with our actual essence. However, by using way of dedicating time and effort to self-exploration and self-interest, we're capable of reconnect with our inner knowledge and live a lifestyles of authenticity and success.

So, whether or not or now not you're a pro practitioner of Kriya Yoga or someone who's simply starting to find out the course of self-discovery, recognizing and embracing your actual self is a transformative and empowering journey that awaits you. Start through placing aside quiet moments for self-contemplated photograph and meditation, and allow the facts of your right self to manual you toward self-attention and a life packed with cause and joy.

Experiencing Oneness and Unity with All

In the good sized realm of spiritual practices, few are as profound and transformative as Kriya Yoga. This historic yogic method gives a effective course in the course of self-cognizance, guiding seekers on a journey of internal awakening and uniting them with the divine essence that is living within. At the coronary heart of Kriya Yoga lies the profound revel in of oneness and group spirit with all.

In the hustle and bustle of our every day lives, it is easy to lose sight of the interconnectedness that exists among ourselves and the sector round us. We end up so engrossed in our man or woman struggles and goals that we neglect about the inherent cohesion that binds us all together. Kriya Yoga serves as a slight reminder, a guiding moderate that illuminates the path in the direction of experiencing this deep connection with all of introduction.

Through the workout of Kriya Yoga, seekers learn how to transcend the guidelines in their physical our bodies and faucet into the huge reservoir of spiritual power that flows inside. As the breath turns into synchronized with the movement of prana, the existence force energy, a profound experience of concord begins to emerge. The practitioner starts offevolved offevolved to comprehend that they may be not spoil away the place however an vital a part of it.

Within this country of oneness, the limits that divide us dissolve, and a deep sense of interconnectedness takes preserve. The seeker becomes acutely conscious that every movement, idea, and emotion reverberates via the complex net of lifestyles. They understand that their personal nicely-being is intricately tied to the properly-being of others, and that with the beneficial resource of uplifting themselves, they make contributions to the upliftment of all.

This enjoy of harmony and oneness isn't just restrained to the individual, however expands to embody all of creation. The seeker starts offevolved to appearance the divine essence that permeates each particle of life, recognizing that all beings are interconnected and part of the equal widespread consciousness. This consciousness fosters a deep feel of compassion, love, and understand for all existence paperwork, essential to a harmonious coexistence with the region spherical us.

In a global regularly marked through department, warfare, and separation, Kriya Yoga gives a transformative direction towards team spirit and oneness. It reminds us that at our middle, we are all related, and that with the aid of embracing this truth, we are able to create a extra compassionate and harmonious international. Through the workout of Kriya Yoga, each seeker has the functionality to enjoy the profound splendor of oneness and crew spirit with all.

Surrendering to the Divine Will

In the route of Kriya Yoga, one of the critical teachings is the concept of surrendering to the Divine Will. This idea holds titanic importance for every seeker on the journey in the path of self-recognition. Whether you've got were given honestly released into the direction of Kriya Yoga or had been schooling it for years, surrendering to the Divine Will is a essential trouble to understand and combine into your non secular workout.

Surrendering to the Divine Will does now not endorse giving up your personal electricity or free will. On the contrary, it is about aligning your will with the better energy, the Divine, and recognizing that there may be a more plan unfolding inside the universe. It is an act of acknowledging that there is a guiding strain past our limited records and trusting in its statistics.

When we give up to the Divine Will, we allow cross of our attachments, dreams, and expectations. We launch the need to control every issue of our lives and alternatively, cultivate a deep feel of faith and surrender. This surrender is not passive; it calls for active participation and a willingness to permit pass of our ego-pushed dreams.

By surrendering to the Divine Will, we open ourselves to divine steerage and allow ourselves to be led in the direction of our most capability. We let bypass of the burden of choice-making and as a substitute, keep in mind that the universe will guide us within the course of the maximum appropriate direction for our boom and evolution.

Surrendering to the Divine Will also enables us cultivate a kingdom of inner peace and contentment. When we surrender to face as lots because the herbal glide of life and give up our desires to the Divine, we discover ourselves in a kingdom of harmony with the universe. We learn how to take transport of and consist of a few element lifestyles gives to us, recognizing that it's miles all part of a grand cosmic plan.

In the workout of Kriya Yoga, surrendering to the Divine Will is an vital step in the direction of self-interest. Through everyday meditation and deep introspection, we learn how to detach ourselves from the illusion of manage and give up to the higher strength interior us. It is thru this give up that we can enjoy the profound union with the Divine and find out our proper nature.

To actually understand and embody the concept of surrendering to the Divine Will, it's far important to domesticate a every day religious exercise. Through regular meditation, breathwork, and self-reflected picture, we are able to step by step permit flow of our attachments, fears, and desires. This workout enables us increase a deeper reference to the Divine and give up our character will to the greater will of the universe.

In prevent, surrendering to the Divine Will is a transformative factor of the journey towards self-popularity in Kriya Yoga. It is ready aligning our will with the better energy and trusting in the know-how of the universe. By surrendering, we domesticate internal peace, contentment, and open ourselves to divine guidance. Through normal workout and deep introspection, we are able to embody this surrender and enjoy the profound union with the Divine.

Living a Life of Purpose and Service

In the historic exercise of Kriya Yoga, the last purpose is self-recognition and union with the divine. However, the adventure in the direction of self-recognition isn't clearly an individual pursuit; it's also approximately dwelling a life of reason and provider to others. This subchapter explores the importance of essential a lifestyles of cause and issuer and the way it complements the exercise of Kriya Yoga for virtually every body.

Living a existence of motive manner aligning our moves, thoughts, and intentions with our private values and aspirations. It requires us to have a clean data of who we're and what we need to make a contribution to the area. By cultivating this revel in of purpose, we're able to deliver extra meaning and success into our lives. Kriya Yoga offers a effective framework for discovering our reason by way of the usage of connecting us to our inner records and guiding us in the direction of serving the pleasant well.

Service is an vital thing of Kriya Yoga, as it allows us to transport past our egoic dispositions and shift our focus closer to the nicely-being of others. It encourages us to growth our love, compassion, and assist to the ones in need. Service can take severa paperwork, from volunteering in our nearby organizations to imparting our skills and apprehend-how to uplift others. By mission selfless agency, we no longer simplest make contributions to the betterment of society but additionally deepen our religious exercise.

Chapter 9: The Philosophy Of Kriya Yoga

Unveiling the Principles of Kriya Yoga

Kriya Yoga: Finding Inner Stillness in a Chaotic World is a profound ebook that delves into the historical exercising of Kriya Yoga, offering insights and steering to people searching out internal peace and spiritual increase. In this subchapter, "Unveiling the Principles of Kriya Yoga," we discover the critical standards that shape the inspiration of this transformative practice.

Kriya Yoga is a manner that mixes breath control, meditation, and self-discipline to evoke the dormant non secular strength interior every character. It is a direction that consequences in self-interest and connects us to the divine essence within us and the universe. Although rooted in historic traditions, Kriya Yoga is offered to everyone, regardless of their non secular or cultural records.

The first principle of Kriya Yoga is the know-how that we are not sincerely bodily beings but moreover spiritual entities. By recognizing and nourishing our non secular nature, we can move beyond the policies of the physical international and enjoy profound states of focus.

The second principle emphasizes the importance of breath control or Pranayama. Through unique respiration techniques, we discover ways to regulate our life strain electricity, moreover known as Prana. By reading the breath, we will harmonize our body, thoughts, and spirit, number one to more potent interest, readability, and commonplace nicely-being.

Another vital precept of Kriya Yoga is the exercising of meditation. Through regular meditation, we domesticate a deep enjoy of inner stillness and silence. This permits us to hook up with our right selves and get proper of get entry to to higher states of attention, leading to progressed self-interest, instinct, and a experience of solidarity with all introduction.

Self-subject is a vital factor of Kriya Yoga. It requires dedication, consistency, and strength of will to the practice. By cultivating energy of will, we expand the ability to manipulate our thoughts, feelings, and movements, most critical to a more balanced and great life.

The very last principle of Kriya Yoga is surrendering to the divine will. As we improvement on our religious adventure, we discover ways to allow skip of our egos and don't forget within the records and steerage of the universe. This give up permits us to align ourselves with the divine drift and revel in a deep sense of peace and achievement.

In stop, "Unveiling the Principles of Kriya Yoga" affords a complete understanding of the middle ideas that underpin this ancient exercise. By incorporating the ones thoughts into our lives, we can embark on a transformative journey of self-discovery, internal stillness, and non secular increase. Whether you are a newbie or an experienced practitioner of Kriya Yoga, this subchapter offers valuable insights and steering that will help you find out internal peace in a chaotic global.

The Concept of Oneness in Kriya Yoga

In the massive expanse of non secular practices, Kriya Yoga stands out as a profound and transformative direction towards self-awareness. Rooted in historic yogic traditions, Kriya Yoga gives a totally unique way to find out inner stillness amidst the chaos of the contemporary-day worldwide. One of the essential necessities inside Kriya Yoga is the concept of oneness.

Oneness, or team spirit attention, is the realization that all beings and the whole universe are interconnected. It is the know-how that we are not ruin away the world round us, however as an opportunity an important part of it. In Kriya Yoga, this idea of oneness is emphasised as a key to unlocking the real potential of our religious journey.

When we apprehend the interconnectedness of all existence, we begin to see beyond the illusions of separation and duality. We recognize that our mind, moves, and energies have an impact no longer most effective on ourselves however additionally at the collective recognition. This awareness cultivates a deep experience of duty and compassion inside the direction of all beings.

Kriya Yoga gives particular techniques and practices that help us enjoy this oneness without delay. Through breath manage, meditation, and self-inquiry, we can get right of get entry to to higher states of interest where the limits amongst ourselves and the sector dissolve. In those moments of profound stillness, we're capable of faucet into the same old electricity that flows thru all beings, identifying our inherent brotherly love with the divine.

The idea of oneness in Kriya Yoga goes beyond intellectual statistics. It is a lived enjoy that transforms the manner we understand ourselves and the area. As we deepen our exercise, we begin to see the inherent divinity in absolutely everyone, each creature, and every detail of creation. We increase a profound sense of love, compassion, and interconnectedness that transcends all obstacles.

The practice of Kriya Yoga is not constrained to a particular institution or belief machine. It is a direction that may be embraced thru all and sundry, irrespective of their records or non secular inclination. The concept of oneness in Kriya Yoga is regular, appealing to the innate preference for unity and connection this is dwelling inside absolutely everyone.

In a worldwide that regularly emphasizes department and separation, the concept of oneness in Kriya Yoga offers a transformative possibility. It invites us to look beyond our versions and understand the underlying harmony that connects us all. Through the exercise of Kriya Yoga, we're capable of domesticate a deep revel in of internal stillness even as embracing the oneness that holds the ability to heal ourselves and the arena.

Incorporating Mindfulness in Kriya Yoga Practice

In the fast-paced and chaotic worldwide we live in, finding internal stillness and peace can often seem like an not possible challenge. However, Kriya Yoga gives a path to attaining this elusive usa of tranquility. Rooted in historical yogic traditions, Kriya Yoga is a effective exercising that combines breath manipulate, meditation, and self-recognition strategies to assist individuals hook up with their inner selves and experience a profound feel of peace and concord.

One of the crucial component elements that could extensively enhance the exercising of Kriya Yoga is the incorporation of mindfulness. Mindfulness, truely placed, is the exercise of being absolutely gift within the 2nd, with out judgment, and with an mind-set of kindness and hobby. It involves being attentive to one's thoughts, feelings, and bodily sensations, and cultivating a deep reputation of the existing 2nd.

By incorporating mindfulness into their Kriya Yoga workout, practitioners can deepen their connection with their internal selves and experience a heightened revel in of awareness. Mindfulness allows human beings to have a observe their thoughts, feelings, and bodily sensations without getting stuck up in them or reacting all at once. This non-reactive stance allows domesticate a experience of detachment and equanimity, allowing humans to navigate thru life's challenges with greater ease and fashion.

Incorporating mindfulness in Kriya Yoga exercise furthermore lets in human beings growth a deeper understanding of their very own minds and concept patterns. By watching their thoughts and emotions with a non-judgmental mind-set, humans can gain insights into the workings in their very own minds and find deep-rooted sorts of questioning and behavior. This self-popularity is a effective tool for non-public increase and transformation, because it allows humans to interrupt free from proscribing ideals and conduct that no longer serve them.

Moreover, mindfulness in Kriya Yoga exercise can beautify the enjoy of meditation. By bringing conscious interest to the breath and the sensations in the frame during meditation, individuals can anchor their attention inside the present second, making it less tough to allow go of distractions and input a country of deep rest and stillness.

In end, incorporating mindfulness in Kriya Yoga exercise offers numerous advantages for people searching for inner stillness in a chaotic international. By cultivating mindfulness, practitioners can deepen their connection with their inner selves, amplify self-reputation, and enhance their meditation practice. Whether you are a seasoned yogi or a newbie on the path of self-discovery, integrating mindfulness into your Kriya Yoga exercise may be a transformative journey within the course of finding inner peace and concord for your existence.

Cultivating Self-Discipline via Kriya Yoga

Self-concern is a different feature which could rework our lives, allowing us to acquire our goals and find out internal stillness amidst the chaos of the arena. Kriya Yoga, a powerful religious workout, gives a path to expand and nurture this crucial fine internal us. By embracing the principles and techniques of Kriya Yoga, everyone can harness their inner strength and cultivate power of will.

At its middle, Kriya Yoga is a holistic technique to self-recognition, integrating physical, intellectual, and non secular dimensions. Through a aggregate of breath manipulate, meditation, and self-meditated picture, Kriya Yoga practitioners discover ways to channel their energies, interest their minds, and align their movements with their maximum purpose. This approach simply ends inside the improvement of energy of mind.

One of the primary motives Kriya Yoga is strong in cultivating self-discipline is its emphasis on ordinary exercise. Practicing Kriya Yoga requires determination and consistency. By assignment each day sadhana (religious exercising), human beings regularly increase a strong feel of dedication and area. Regularity in workout strengthens the energy of thoughts, enabling practitioners to stay centered and persevere despite the fact that confronted with worrying conditions or distractions.

Furthermore, Kriya Yoga teaches us to have a look at our thoughts, feelings, and actions with out judgment. This self-attention is a vital component of growing energy of will. By becoming greater privy to our behavior and inclinations, we benefit the functionality to consciously pick out our responses in vicinity of reacting all of sudden. Through the exercising of Kriya Yoga, we cultivate the strength to overcome our desires and impulses, making alternatives that align with our better aspirations.

Kriya Yoga moreover promotes the cultivation of virtues along side endurance, willpower, and perseverance. These skills are critical in retaining self-control. As we improvement in our exercising, we encounter severa barriers and setbacks. However, through the classes of Kriya Yoga, we discover ways to view the ones annoying situations as possibilities for increase and self-development. By persevering thru troubles and staying committed to our practice, we growth an unwavering treatment and unwavering energy of will.

Chapter 10: The Science Of Kriya Yoga

The Breath: Key to Inner Stillness

In the fast-paced and chaotic global we live in, locating inner stillness can experience like an elusive aim. However, there's a powerful tool that may assist us navigate through the chaos and discover a revel in of peace within ourselves – the breath. In the workout of Kriya Yoga, the breath performs a widespread role in accomplishing internal stillness and experiencing a deeper connection with our actual selves.

The breath isn't always simplest a physical feature that keeps us alive; it is a gateway to our internal global. When we bring our interest to the breath, we grow to be privy to the prevailing second and domesticate a kingdom of mindfulness. This easy act of aware respiratory lets in us to permit glide of problems approximately the past or destiny and brings us into the proper here and now.

In Kriya Yoga, specific breathing strategies, called pranayama, are hired to harness the strength of the breath. Through the ones strategies, we learn how to manipulate and direct the flow of prana, or lifestyles strain electricity, interior our bodies. This permits us to stability our electricity facilities, or chakras, and harmonize our bodily, highbrow, and non secular factors.

Practicing pranayama no longer best brings us physical blessings, together with progressed lung capability and oxygenation, but it also lets in to calm the thoughts and decrease strain. As we consciously modify our breath, we spark off the parasympathetic stressful machine, triggering the rest reaction and promoting a kingdom of inner stillness.

By incorporating pranayama into our every day normal, we are able to revel in a profound transformation in our lives. As we grow to be greater attuned to our breath, we increase a heightened experience of self-consciousness and advantage more control over our mind and feelings. We begin to understand the varieties of our thoughts and might choose to answer in area of react to outside activities.

Furthermore, the breath becomes a bridge that connects us to our spiritual essence. As we deepen our breath and extend our focus, we open ourselves as a good deal as the possibility of experiencing profound states of meditation and non secular awakening. The breath becomes a automobile for accessing the depths of our being and connecting with the divine.

In surrender, the breath is a effective tool that may assist us find inner stillness in a chaotic global. Through the exercise of Kriya Yoga and pranayama, we are able to harness the transformative strength of the breath and revel in a deeper reference to ourselves and the universe. By incorporating those practices into our each day lives, we will navigate through the traumatic conditions of life with grace and cultivate a sense of peace that transcends the external turmoil.

Understanding Prana and Pranayama

In the historical yogic subculture, the idea of Prana and Pranayama holds extremely good importance. Prana, frequently referred to as the lifestyles pressure energy, is the diffused power that permeates the whole lot in the universe. It is the crucial pressure that sustains all living beings and is answerable for our physical, intellectual, and spiritual well-being. Pranayama, on the other hand, is the exercising of controlling and harnessing this existence pressure electricity for our ordinary boom and transformation.

For all people, whether or now not or no longer you are a amateur or an advanced practitioner of Kriya Yoga, know-how Prana and Pranayama is important. By statistics and working with those necessities, we're capable of faucet into the infinite capability that lies inner us and experience a profound sense of internal stillness amidst the chaos of the arena.

Prana isn't virtually the breath we take; it's far masses extra than that. It is the power that flows via severa channels in our diffused body, called Nadis. These Nadis are interconnected and shape a complicated network, just like the circulatory system. When the flow of Prana is smooth and unobstructed, we revel in colourful health, readability of mind, and a deep revel in of internal peace. However, at the same time as the glide of Prana is blocked or imbalanced, it may show up as physical or highbrow illnesses.

Pranayama, which interprets to "boom of lifestyles strain strength," is a effective device to balance and purify our Pranic strength. Through unique respiration strategies, we're capable of regulate the waft of Prana, cleanse the Nadis, and awaken our dormant non secular capacity. Regular exercise of Pranayama not best allows in improving our bodily health however additionally complements our highbrow clarity and spiritual recognition.

For the ones engaged within the exercising of Kriya Yoga, Pranayama becomes an critical a part of their sadhana (spiritual workout). It prepares the practitioner for better states of reputation and aids in the journey within the direction of self-consciousness. By consciously walking with the breath, you may although cultivate a deep connection with the subtle nation-states of lifestyles and revel in the profound stillness that lies beyond the fluctuations of the thoughts.

Whether you're new to Kriya Yoga or have been at the route for some time, knowledge Prana and Pranayama is essential for your boom and evolution. Through the exercising of Pranayama, you can harness the electricity of Prana and embark on a transformative journey toward internal stillness and self-discovery. So, permit us to dive deeper into the region of Prana and find out the captivating global of Pranayama, in which the breath turns into a gateway to our right essence.

Exploring the Chakras in Kriya Yoga

In the historical workout of Kriya Yoga, the concept of chakras holds a splendid vicinity. These energy facilities are believed to exist inside our diffused frame and play a crucial role in our physical, intellectual, and non secular properly-being. Understanding and exploring the chakras in Kriya Yoga can help us free up our internal functionality, discover stability, and hook up with a higher cognizance.

The word "chakra" comes from the Sanskrit language and translates to "wheel" or "disk." It refers back to the spinning vortexes of strength which may be positioned along the spine, from the lowest to the crown of the pinnacle. Each chakra corresponds to specific tendencies and factors of our being, which consist of physical fitness, emotions, intuition, and non secular boom.

In Kriya Yoga, practitioners analyze techniques to set off and harmonize those chakras, permitting the unfastened flow of energy in the course of the body. This approach lets in to remove blockages and restore stability, most crucial to a country of inner stillness and reference to the Divine.

The e-book "Kriya Yoga: Finding Inner Stillness in a Chaotic World" delves into the exploration of the chakras in Kriya Yoga, presenting practical guidance and insights for practitioners of all degrees. It offers a entire knowledge of each chakra, its features, and the techniques used to rouse and balance them.

Through slight moves, breathwork, meditation, and visualization, Kriya Yoga practitioners can prompt and purify the chakras, permitting them to characteristic optimally. This alignment of the chakras promotes bodily strength, emotional balance, intellectual readability, and non secular awakening.

The subchapter on exploring the chakras in Kriya Yoga offers step-with the useful useful resource of-step instructions, guided meditations, and personal anecdotes to assist readers of their journey. It emphasizes the significance of self-focus, self-care, and normal workout to revel in the transformative electricity of the chakras.

Whether you're new to Kriya Yoga or an professional practitioner, this subchapter is a treasured beneficial resource to deepen your statistics of the chakras and decorate your ordinary well-being. It offers a roadmap to discover and wake up the subtle electricity facilities, essential to a greater experience of harmony, peace, and spiritual increase.

Embark on this adventure of self-discovery and tap into the countless potential inside you. Explore the chakras in Kriya Yoga and enjoy the profound transformation that awaits you at the direction to internal stillness in a chaotic worldwide.

Harnessing the Power of Kundalini Energy

Kriya Yoga: Finding Inner Stillness in a Chaotic World

Understanding Kundalini Energy:

Kundalini is regularly represented as a coiled serpent, mendacity dormant at the lowest of the spine. It is considered the divine cosmic power that holds large functionality for non secular awakening. When wakened, Kundalini ascends through the power facilities alongside the spine, called chakras, bringing about a heightened u . S . A . Of interest and inner transformation. This electricity is said to be the supply of our energy, creativity, and spiritual enlightenment.

Awakening Kundalini:

The workout of Kriya Yoga is an powerful way to evoke the dormant Kundalini strength. Through a aggregate of breathwork, meditation, and precise techniques, Kriya Yoga practitioners can step by step awaken and direct this effective energy. Kriya Yoga strategies purify the nadis (power channels) and do away with blockages, allowing the Kundalini to upward thrust actually and harmoniously.

Benefits of Harnessing Kundalini Energy:

Harnessing Kundalini strength offers numerous benefits for human beings on the direction of Kriya Yoga and beyond. It brings approximately a deep experience of inner stillness, clarity, and reference to the divine. As Kundalini ascends, it complements our bodily and highbrow well-being, boosts creativity and intuition, and deepens our spiritual reviews. Kundalini strength is also believed to rouse dormant colleges internal us, increasing our recognition and facilitating self-interest.

Precautions and Guidance:

As Kundalini energy is immensely effective, it is vital to technique its awakening with warning and under the guidance of an professional Kriya Yoga trainer. Due to its depth, it's miles essential to prepare oneself bodily, mentally, and emotionally for this journey. Regular exercise, location, and a balanced manner of existence are key factors in harnessing Kundalini electricity safely and efficiently.

Chapter 11: Step-By Way Of-Step Guide To Kriya Yoga Practice

Preparing the Body and Mind for Kriya Yoga

Before embarking at the transformative adventure of Kriya Yoga, it is crucial to put together every the frame and mind. This subchapter objectives to manual all people inquisitive about Kriya Yoga, irrespective of their level of enjoy, on a way to cultivate the right situations for this exercise. Whether you're a pro practitioner or a newbie, the ones preparatory steps will help you delve deeper into the profound stillness and inner peace that Kriya Yoga offers.

Physical Preparation:

To optimize the benefits of Kriya Yoga, it is crucial to hold a healthful frame. Engaging in ordinary physical exercising, which include yoga asanas, can loosen the muscle groups and beautify flexibility, bearing in mind extra ease at some point of meditation. Additionally, incorporating pranayama, the exercise of breath manipulate, can assist purify the frame, increase lung capability, and stimulate strength go together with the go with the flow. Proper nutrients, hydration, and appropriate enough sleep are also crucial to useful resource a sturdy and colourful physical vessel for the practice.

Mental Preparation:

Preparing the mind is in addition crucial for the workout of Kriya Yoga. Cultivating a disciplined and centered attitude is fundamental to navigating the worrying conditions which could rise up in the course of meditation. Regular meditation, even for a few minutes every day, can help train the mind to grow to be more calm, focused, and gift. Exploring mindfulness strategies and incorporating them into each day sports activities can similarly enhance mental clarity and recognition.

Emotional Preparation:

Emotional well-being performs a first-rate function in Kriya Yoga. It is vital to create a safe and nurturing environment for oneself, every internally and externally. Practicing self-compassion, forgiveness, and gratitude can assist launch emotional tensions and domesticate a nice mind-set. Engaging in activities that carry satisfaction and fulfillment can also make a contribution to emotional stability and normal nicely-being.

Creating Sacred Space:

Setting up a committed vicinity for exercise can considerably beautify the effectiveness of Kriya Yoga. Designating a quiet and clutter-loose place, free from distractions, allows for a deeper connection with the exercising. Personalizing the gap with sacred devices, collectively with candles, incense, or pics that inspire and uplift, can create a serene ecosystem conducive to meditation.

Asanas: The Physical Aspect of Kriya Yoga

In the journey of self-discovery and religious growth, Kriya Yoga offers a holistic technique that encompasses numerous additives of our being. One of the essential pillars of this ancient exercise is Asanas, which focus on the physical detail of Kriya Yoga. Asanas, or yoga postures, play a critical feature in harmonizing the body, thoughts, and spirit, allowing practitioners to find inner stillness inside the midst of a chaotic worldwide.

In Kriya Yoga, Asanas are not absolutely bodily sporting sports; they'll be a manner to awaken and energize the subtle electricity centers within the body, known as chakras. By training a sequence of postures, people can channel their power and attain a rustic of stability and power. These postures are designed to boom flexibility, electricity, and enhance the waft of prana (life pressure strength) at some degree within the body.

The workout of Asanas in Kriya Yoga offers severa advantages for each person, regardless of age, physical fitness, or revel in. Regular exercise facilitates in enhancing physical health via developing regular flexibility, toning muscles, and enhancing posture. It moreover aids in relieving pressure, decreasing anxiety, and selling intellectual readability and awareness. Asanas help release anxiety and pollution from the body, growing a feel of rejuvenation and electricity.

For the ones mainly interested in Kriya Yoga, Asanas serve as a preparation for deeper practices, collectively with pranayama (respiratory strategies) and meditation. The physical postures assist to purify and guide the body, making it more receptive to the diffused energies and higher states of recognition that Kriya Yoga dreams to attain. Asanas are like a bridge that connects the physical realm with the spiritual realm, permitting practitioners to experience the profound connection among frame, thoughts, and spirit.

It is critical to approach the workout of Asanas with mindfulness and apprehend for one's frame. Each person's frame is specific, and it is vital to pay attention to its barriers and honor them. It is not about attaining exceptional poses but as an opportunity approximately cultivating consciousness and reputation of 1's frame and its capabilities. With regular workout and staying power, development will simply spread.

In give up, Asanas are an vital part of Kriya Yoga, presenting a course to physical nicely-being, intellectual readability, and non secular increase. By incorporating those physical postures into our each day lives, we're capable of locate internal stillness and harmony amidst the chaos of the world. Whether you're new to yoga or a pro practitioner, embracing Asanas can offer a profound adventure of self-discovery and transformation.

Pranayama Techniques in Kriya Yoga

In the ancient technological information of yoga, one of the most powerful and transformative practices is the paintings of pranayama. Derived from the Sanskrit words "prana" meaning important existence stress and "ayama" because of this to increase or manipulate, pranayama encompasses various breathing techniques which could profoundly decorate our bodily, intellectual, and religious well-being. In the arena of Kriya Yoga, these pranayama strategies keep a unique area, supplying a pathway to internal stillness and harmony amidst the chaos of the modern global.

Kriya Yoga, a machine of spiritual meditation and self-awareness, emphasizes the aggregate of breath manage with meditation and willpower. The pranayama strategies hired in Kriya Yoga feature a bridge maximum of the physical and non secular dimensions, allowing practitioners to connect to their internal essence and get admission to heightened states of interest. These techniques artwork via regulating the glide of prana, the lifestyles force electricity that permeates our being, and harmonizing its motion all through the body.

One of the essential pranayama techniques in Kriya Yoga is the Ujjayi breath. Characterized with the aid of a gentle constriction of the throat, Ujjayi breath creates a tender, hissing sound that calms the mind and soothes the worried device. This method facilitates to supply reputation to our breath, fostering a deep sense of relaxation and awareness at some stage in meditation.

Another crucial pranayama approach in Kriya Yoga is Nadi Shodhana, or trade nose respiratory. This practice consists of alternating the inhalation and exhalation the various left and right nostrils, balancing the go together with the flow of power in the frame and purifying the subtle electricity channels. Nadi Shodhana cultivates intellectual clarity, reduces strain, and harmonizes the frame-mind complex.

Kriya Yoga additionally carries Kapalabhati, a dynamic respiratory method that consists of fast and forceful exhalations decided with the aid of way of the use of passive inhalations. This exercising now not brilliant cleanses the breathing machine but additionally invigorates the body, complements reputation, and purifies the mind.

By regularly training pranayama techniques in Kriya Yoga, people can enjoy a massive variety of blessings. These encompass reduced stress and tension, stepped forward cognizance and recognition, advanced breathing feature, extended strength degrees, and a deeper connection to their spiritual self. No recall one's statistics or degree of experience, the profound teachings of Kriya Yoga and its pranayama strategies provide a course toward internal stillness, self-discovery, and transformation within the midst of existence's chaos.

In conclusion, the subchapter on Pranayama Techniques in Kriya Yoga highlights the transformative strength of breath control in the exercising of Kriya Yoga. By exploring numerous pranayama strategies which includes Ujjayi breath, Nadi Shodhana, and Kapalabhati, practitioners can release the capability for deep rest, extended reputation, and spiritual growth. Whether you're new to yoga or an experienced practitioner, the ones techniques provide a gateway to locating inner stillness and peace in our speedy-paced and chaotic international.

Meditation and Visualization in Kriya Yoga

In the ancient exercise of Kriya Yoga, meditation and visualization play a crucial feature in attaining internal stillness and peace amidst the chaos of our contemporary-day global. These effective techniques had been exceeded down thru generations, supporting people from all walks of existence to connect to their internal selves and revel in profound spiritual increase.

Meditation lies on the coronary heart of Kriya Yoga, imparting a pathway to go beyond the limitations of the mind and tap into the countless wellspring of reputation within. Through regular meditation exercise, people learn how to quiet the steady chatter of their mind, letting them delve into the depths in their being and connect to their better self.

This kingdom of deep meditation cultivates a experience of inner calmness, clarity, and heightened interest, main to a more fulfilled and beneficial life.

Visualization is any other vital factor of Kriya Yoga, harnessing the power of the thoughts to occur exceptional modifications in a unmarried's life. By visualizing preferred results and memories, humans can create a blueprint for their future and align their intentions with the time-honored energy. Visualization strategies in Kriya Yoga include growing vibrant mental photographs of one's goals, aspirations, or maybe bodily recuperation, allowing the unconscious mind to paintings in the direction of turning those visualizations into reality.

Through the aggregate of meditation and visualization, Kriya Yoga practitioners can faucet into their innate capability and bring about profound transformation on bodily, highbrow, and spiritual stages. The workout of Kriya Yoga permits human beings expand a deeper connection with their right selves, permitting them to navigate the traumatic conditions of lifestyles with extra ease and beauty.

Whether you are a pro yogi or new to the arena of Kriya Yoga, the ones strategies are to be had to every body. Regardless of your age, ancient past, or beliefs, the mind of meditation and visualization can be incorporated into your every day everyday, helping you discover inner stillness and navigate the chaos of the contemporary international.

In the subchapter "Meditation and Visualization in Kriya Yoga," we can discover diverse meditation techniques, beginning from breath-centered meditation to mantra repetition. We can even delve into the artwork of visualization, presenting step-thru the use of-step steering on the manner to create and take area your desires thru the electricity of the thoughts.

Chapter 12: Integrating Kriya Yoga Into Daily Life

Applying Kriya Yoga Principles to Relationships

In the adventure of lifestyles, relationships keep an essential location. Whether it is our bond with own family, friends, or romantic partners, they play a widespread function in shaping our studies and common properly-being. Kriya Yoga, a profound spiritual exercise, gives precious thoughts that may beautify our relationships and convey harmony and love into our lives.

At its center, Kriya Yoga is a route inside the path of self-recognition and inner stillness. It emphasizes the relationship between the character soul and the divine attention. By making use of those necessities to our relationships, we are able to cultivate a deeper facts, compassion, and love for others.

One of the essential standards of Kriya Yoga is self-awareness. By cultivating self-attention, we turn out to be greater attuned to our mind, emotions, and actions. This heightened interest permits us to recognize and apprehend our very personal patterns and triggers within relationships. With this facts, we are able to consciously pick to answer in preference to react, fundamental to extra healthy and extra harmonious interactions.

Another critical principle is non-attachment. Kriya Yoga teaches us to detach ourselves from the outcomes and expectancies we often impose on our relationships. By surrendering the want for manage, we permit the glide of love and compassion to manual our interactions. This exercise prevents us from becoming entangled in vain conflicts and fosters a revel in of freedom and reputation internal our relationships.

Kriya Yoga also emphasizes the energy of forgiveness. Holding onto grudges and beyond hurts best creates limitations to love and connection. By working within the course of forgiveness, we launch ourselves from the burden of resentment and open ourselves as lots as recovery and increase. Forgiveness allows us to create area for romance and information to flourish interior our relationships.

Furthermore, Kriya Yoga teaches us the importance of stability. In relationships, it's miles important to discover a balance amongst giving and receiving, among our very private wishes and the needs of others. By locating this equilibrium, we create an surroundings in which both people can thrive and make contributions to the relationship's increase.

In stop, utilising Kriya Yoga thoughts to our relationships can supply profound alterations. By cultivating self-attention, walking toward non-attachment, embracing forgiveness, and searching for stability, we create a foundation of love, records, and harmony interior our connections. Kriya Yoga gives us the tools to navigate the complexities of relationships with grace and compassion, ultimately allowing us to find out inner stillness in a chaotic international.

Finding Inner Stillness amidst Work and Responsibilities

In current rapid-paced and demanding international, locating inner stillness can look like an elusive intention. We are constantly bombarded with paintings duties, closing dates, and the in no way-completing goals of each day life. However, amidst the chaos, there can be a powerful device that may assist us discover tranquility and peace – Kriya Yoga.

Kriya Yoga is an historical practice that offers a pathway to internal stillness and self-hobby. It offers a scientific technique to harmonizing the frame, mind, and spirit, allowing human beings to navigate the worrying conditions of existence effortlessly and style. Whether you are a seasoned practitioner or new to the world of yoga, Kriya Yoga offers a completely particular set of strategies that may be protected into your every day recurring.

One of the essential factor thoughts of Kriya Yoga is the mixture of breath control and meditation. By consciously regulating our breath, we are able to calm the thoughts and create a feel of inner stillness. Through unique respiratory techniques, together with alternate nostril breathing or ujjayi breath, we will set off the parasympathetic worrying gadget, inducing a country of deep rest.

Integrating Kriya Yoga into our busy lives requires determination and location. It is essential to carve out dedicated time each day to workout those strategies. Even a couple of minutes of targeted respiratory and meditation may also additionally have a profound impact on our regular well-being. By prioritizing our inner stillness, we end up more green and efficient in our art work and duties.

Moreover, Kriya Yoga teaches us to detach from the outcomes of our movements. It reminds us that we are not described via way of our artwork or obligations however through using the essence of who we're. This facts permits us to method our responsibilities with a experience of detachment and equanimity, decreasing stress and tension.

As we delve deeper into the exercise of Kriya Yoga, we start to domesticate a revel in of inner peace that is unshakable. We learn how to find out stillness amidst the chaos, developing a sanctuary inside ourselves. This inner sanctuary turns into our secure haven at some point of tough times, allowing us to navigate through existence's u.S.And downs with grace and resilience.

In give up, Kriya Yoga gives a effective tool for finding inner stillness amidst the goals of exertions and duties. By integrating breath manipulate, meditation, and detachment into our every day lives, we will cultivate a experience of tranquility and peace. Whether you're new to Kriya Yoga or a pro practitioner, incorporating those techniques into your regular can redesign your experience of life.

Embrace the workout of Kriya Yoga and embark on a adventure of self-discovery and inner serenity inside the midst of a chaotic global.

Kriya Yoga as a Tool for Emotional Balance

In cutting-edge fast-paced and chaotic international, finding inner stillness and emotional stability has emerge as increasingly more tough for anyone. The ordinary bombardment of statistics, strain, and obligations can take a toll on our intellectual and emotional nicely-being. However, there can be a effective tool that could assist us navigate via those demanding situations and find out a enjoy of calm amidst the chaos – Kriya Yoga.

Kriya Yoga is an historical exercising that originated in India and has been exceeded down thru generations of yogis. It is a holistic approach to non secular development that combines breath manipulate, meditation, and willpower. While Kriya Yoga is deeply rooted in spirituality, its advantages increase a ways past the world of religion or notion structures. It is a workout that can be embraced through anybody, irrespective of their ancient beyond or beliefs.

One of the important thing blessings of running closer to Kriya Yoga is its functionality to cultivate emotional balance. Through the workout of controlled respiratory strategies, called pranayama, we discover ways to regulate the go with the flow of electricity in our our our bodies. This allows us to launch pent-up feelings and find a harmonious balance within ourselves. By consciously directing our breath, we will allow pass of stress, tension, and negativity, changing them with emotions of peace, joy, and quietness.

Moreover, Kriya Yoga teaches us to study our mind and emotions without judgment or attachment. Through ordinary meditation workout, we increase a heightened hobby of our internal panorama. This interest lets in us to detach from our feelings, permitting them to stand up and bypass without becoming beaten or controlled thru them. We discover ways to reply to lifestyles's stressful conditions with equanimity, in desire to reacting swiftly or being over excited through our emotions.

Additionally, the workout of Kriya Yoga facilitates us reconnect with our inner selves, fostering self-love and reputation. As we delve deeper into our exercising, we enlarge a extra understanding of our emotions and their underlying reasons. This self-reflected photograph and introspection permit us to increase compassion inside the path of ourselves and others, fundamental to improved relationships and a greater experience of desired well-being.

In stop, Kriya Yoga is a precious tool for reaching emotional balance in cutting-edge chaotic worldwide. By incorporating breath control, meditation, and strength of mind into our every day lives, we will domesticate a sense of inner stillness and discover peace amidst the turmoil. Whether you are new to yoga or a seasoned practitioner, Kriya Yoga offers a transformative path within the route of emotional properly-being for absolutely everyone.

Cultivating a Spirit of Service via Kriya Yoga

In the workout of Kriya Yoga, one in each of its maximum profound teachings is the significance of cultivating a spirit of service. This ancient yogic culture no longer high-quality offers a path to internal stillness and self-focus however furthermore encourages people to increase their practice beyond themselves and into the area. Through selfless carrier, practitioners of Kriya Yoga should make a fine effect on others and find a deeper revel in of fulfillment and purpose of their lives.

Kriya Yoga teaches us that right spirituality is not entirely about personal increase and enlightenment however furthermore about recognizing our interconnectedness with all beings. By cultivating a spirit of service, we well known that we're a part of a larger complete and feature a responsibility to contribute to the nicely-being of others. This statistics is on the coronary heart of Kriya Yoga's teachings on seva, or selfless service.

Service can take many paperwork, each massive and small. It may be as clean as providing a supporting hand to a neighbor in need or volunteering at a community charity. It also can contain dedicating one's capabilities and abilities to a reason that aligns with one's values and passions. Through provider, we have got got the opportunity to hold love, compassion, and restoration to those who are suffering and in want.

Kriya Yoga emphasizes that issuer ought to be finished with none expectation of reward or popularity. It isn't about searching out validation or boosting our ego but as an opportunity about acting from a place of real compassion and empathy. When we serve others selflessly, we tap into the innate goodness interior us and revel in a profound experience of satisfaction and achievement.

Furthermore, the exercise of Kriya Yoga itself may be visible as a form of service. By dedicating ourselves to our non secular boom and inner transformation, we become beacons of mild and notion for others. Our very personal journey inside the direction of self-recognition can encourage and uplift those spherical us, spreading positivity and peace in the international.

In give up, cultivating a spirit of company thru Kriya Yoga is a powerful manner to deepen our workout and contribute to the nicely-being of others. By selflessly serving others, we now not most effective make a high-quality effect on the area but moreover enjoy a profound experience of pleasure and reason. Through acts of provider, large or small, we are able to supply love, compassion, and recuperation to the ones in need and inspire others on their personal religious direction. Let us encompass the classes of

Kriya Yoga and embark on a journey of selfless carrier, fostering a global full of kindness, cohesion, and concord.

Chapter 13: Advanced Practices And Techniques

Exploring Higher States of Consciousness

In the search for internal stillness, seekers frequently find themselves craving to explore higher states of hobby. These extended states hold the promise of profound insights, non secular boom, and an accelerated understanding of truth. One such path that results in the ones wonderful states is Kriya Yoga.

Kriya Yoga, an historical practice rooted inside the teachings of the exceptional yogis of India, gives a scientific technique to unlocking the capability of the human thoughts and spirit. It is a course that transcends religious limitations and is available to everybody, irrespective of their historical past or ideals.

At the coronary coronary heart of Kriya Yoga lies the idea of higher states of attention. These states may be described as altered states of attention wherein the practitioner evaluations a heightened enjoy of reference to the divine, a deep experience of internal peace, and a profound information of the character of reality.

Through a aggregate of breath manipulate, meditation, and specific techniques, Kriya Yoga practitioners are able to spark off dormant energies internal themselves, allowing them to faucet into those higher states. As the mind becomes however and the senses are withdrawn, the practitioner enters a country of accelerated attention, transcending the restrictions of the physical global.

In the ones prolonged states, practitioners often file experiencing a deep revel in of interconnectedness with all residing beings. They may moreover benefit insights into the person of life and the real purpose of existence. Many describe a enjoy of being guided through a higher strength or divine intelligence, most important them in the direction of self-recognition and religious awakening.

The exploration of better states of cognizance thru Kriya Yoga now not most effective brings personal transformation however furthermore has the capability to genuinely effect the world round us. As people turn out to be more attuned to their real nature and the interconnectedness of all subjects, they're evidently willing to act with compassion, love, and facts. This ripple impact can result in profound modifications inside the lives of those they contact, developing a extra harmonious and compassionate world.

Whether you're new to Kriya Yoga or have been on the path for years, the exploration of higher states of awareness is a transformative adventure that awaits. Through devoted exercise, an open mind, and a sincere coronary coronary heart, you could delve into the depths of your being and find out the endless functionality that lies interior. Embark on this adventure, and discover the profound stillness and knowledge that appearance in advance to you in the better geographical areas of hobby through the exercise of Kriya Yoga.

Deepening Meditation through Advanced Techniques

In the historic workout of Kriya Yoga, the journey of self-discovery and internal stillness is an ongoing device. As practitioners delve deeper into their meditation workout, they embark on a course of self-popularity and transcendence. This subchapter explores the advanced strategies that can take your meditation exercise to new heights, permitting you to faucet into the profound peace and readability that lies inner.

One superior method that could deepen your meditation exercise is the incorporation of pranayama, or breath manipulate. Pranayama strategies, which includes trade nostril respiratory and breath retention, assist to modify the go together with the drift of power within the body and calm the mind. By focusing on the breath, practitioners can gain a rustic of deep rest and heightened attention, facilitating a profound connection with their internal selves.

Another technique to beautify your meditation exercise is the usage of mantras and affirmations. Mantras are effective sounds or terms that could help attention the thoughts and invoke a experience of tranquility. By repeating a mantra or confirmation in the end of meditation, you may quiet the intellectual chatter and domesticate a deep experience of inner peace. Whether it's miles a conventional Sanskrit mantra or a private affirmation, the vibrational power created through these sacred sounds can open the doors to higher states of popularity.

Visualization is however each one-of-a-kind superior method that can be employed to deepen your meditation workout. By visualizing serene and sacred spaces, which includes a non violent lawn or a tranquil ocean, you may create a highbrow sanctuary that lets in for deep rest and focus.

Visualization strategies additionally can be used to hook up with your higher self or divine electricity, allowing you to tap right into a infinite well of reputation and steerage.

Finally, the exercising of mindfulness can extensively decorate your meditation adventure. By cultivating a non-judgmental recognition of the winning second, you may definitely immerse your self within the revel in of meditation. Mindfulness strategies, including frame scans and sensory popularity, will can help you growth a profound feel of presence and stillness, bearing in mind a deeper connection with your internal being.

As you hold your exploration of Kriya Yoga and the transformative energy of meditation, these superior techniques will feature valuable device on your route to inner peace and self-discovery. Remember, the journey of deepening your meditation exercise is precise to all and sundry, so encompass those techniques with an open coronary coronary heart and mind. May your workout bring you ever in the route of locating internal stillness within the midst of a chaotic worldwide.

The Role of Mantras in Kriya Yoga

In the ancient way of existence of Kriya Yoga, mantras play a substantial function in guiding practitioners towards inner stillness and self-focus. Derived from the Sanskrit words "guy" (mind) and "tra" (device), mantras are effective sound vibrations that create a harmonious resonance inside the frame and thoughts. These sacred syllables preserve the crucial component to unlocking the dormant non secular energy that lies inner each person.

Mantras act as a bridge between the outer worldwide and the inner realm of attention. Through the repetition of particular sounds, practitioners are able to pass the restrictions of the rational thoughts and get right of access to higher states of recognition. The vibrations generated via mantras have a transformative impact on the physical, mental, and lively tiers, purifying and aligning the practitioner's being.

Kriya Yoga emphasizes the usage of unique mantras, called bija mantras, which can be seed syllables representing truely one of a type factors of the divine. These mantras are carefully chosen to resonate with the practitioner's character energy and guide them towards self-awareness. By focusing the mind and uttering those sacred sounds, you may although tap into the countless supply of non secular energy and experience profound internal transformation.

The repetition of mantras in Kriya Yoga isn't truely a mechanical exercising however a deeply spiritual exercise. Each mantra holds a completely unique vibrational incredible that awakens specific elements of attention. As the practitioner chants the mantra, the sound reverberates in the body, purifying the energy facilities (chakras) and activating dormant religious schools. This manner permits for the release of blockages and the growth of attention.

Furthermore, mantras in Kriya Yoga feature a focal point for attention and meditation. By directing the mind within the course of a single sound or word, practitioners can regardless of the fact that the fluctuations of thoughts and input a nation of internal stillness. The mantra acts as an anchor, preventing the thoughts from wandering and bringing it lower back to the prevailing 2nd.

While the exercising of mantras in Kriya Yoga is deeply rooted in way of life, it's far available to surely anybody. Regardless of 1's history or spiritual beliefs, the strength of sound vibrations may be harnessed to beautify one's spiritual adventure. The regular repetition of mantras brings approximately a deep experience of peace, readability, and connection to the divine internal.

In end, mantras are an essential part of the Kriya Yoga manner of existence, guiding practitioners within the direction of internal stillness and self-interest. Through the electricity of sacred sound, mantras purify the thoughts, awaken non secular energies, and facilitate deep meditation. By incorporating mantras into our day by day practice, we are capable of locate solace and move past the chaos of the external world, in the end discovering the eternal stillness this is residing within every parents.

Developing Intuition through Kriya Yoga

In the pursuit of locating internal stillness in a chaotic international, Kriya Yoga offers a profound direction in the direction of self-discovery and religious growth. This historical practice not handiest allows us connect to the divine power interior us but moreover enhances our intuitive capabilities, allowing us to navigate lifestyles's disturbing situations with readability and recognition. Through the normal practice of Kriya Yoga, we're capable of expand and sharpen our instinct, starting doors to a deeper know-how of ourselves and the vicinity round us.

Intuition, regularly referred to as our inner voice or intestine feeling, is a powerful device that courses us in the direction of making informed choices and aligning with our right cause. It serves as a compass, steering us in the course of the proper route, even though proper judgment also can appear inadequate. Kriya Yoga gives a framework for cultivating and growing this innate capability.

One of the vital element techniques in which Kriya Yoga enhances intuition is with the aid of way of quieting the thoughts and bringing us proper into a country of deep inner stillness. The exercise involves severa strategies, which includes breath control, meditation, and asanas, which help us detach from the outdoor distractions and connect to our innermost being. As we delve deeper into this country of stillness, we come to be greater attuned to our intuition, permitting it to guide us with greater clarity and accuracy.

Chapter 14: Overcoming Challenges

Dealing with Distractions and Restlessness

In present day speedy-paced and chaotic worldwide, finding internal stillness can be a daunting venture. We are constantly bombarded with distractions that pull us faraway from our dreams and go away us feeling confused and unfulfilled. However, in the exercise of Kriya Yoga, we are able to find out powerful techniques to fight these traumatic situations and discover actual peace and harmony interior ourselves.

Distractions can are available many forms: the consistent buzz of our smartphones, the demands of our busy schedules, or the in no manner-ending pass of mind that occupy our minds. These distractions not simplest prevent our capability to reputation but moreover drain our strength and leave us feeling overwhelmed. Thankfully, Kriya Yoga gives us with powerful device to conquer those barriers.

One of the essential practices of Kriya Yoga is breath manipulate. By studying to modify our breath, we are able to calm our minds and convey our interest decrease again to the prevailing 2nd. Through pranayama strategies, collectively with trade nose respiratory or the breath of fireside, we are capable of launch tension and invite a enjoy of tranquility into our lives. These practices not only help us address distractions however furthermore increase our conventional recognition and hobby.

Another key element of Kriya Yoga is meditation. Through regular meditation, we're capable of train our minds to become plenty tons much less reactive to outdoor stimuli and further focused in our internal being. By looking our thoughts with out judgment and permitting them to bypass with the useful resource of like clouds inside the sky, we are capable of detach ourselves from distractions and cultivate a deep feel of internal stillness. With time and exercising, meditation becomes a safe haven from restlessness, allowing us to find solace amidst the chaos of day by day life.

In addition to breath control and meditation, Kriya Yoga emphasizes the significance of willpower and self-cognizance. By putting clear intentions and growing a balanced ordinary, we are capable of decrease external distractions and create an environment conducive to inner peace. Through normal self-mirrored photo and introspection, we will select out the inspiration causes of our restlessness and increase techniques to address them.

In end, coping with distractions and restlessness is a not unusual struggle for all people in cutting-edge-day speedy-paced global. However, through the practice of Kriya Yoga, we're able to find internal stillness amidst the chaos. By incorporating breath manipulate, meditation, and willpower into our lives, we're able to overcome distractions, domesticate awareness, and experience a deep revel in of peace and harmony inside ourselves. Whether you're new to Kriya Yoga or a seasoned practitioner, those strategies are useful gadget for navigating the disturbing situations of modern-day existence and finding actual achievement.

Navigating Doubts and Inner Resistance

Doubts and inner resistance are common evaluations at the religious course, and practicing Kriya Yoga is not any exception. In this subchapter, we will discover the manner to navigate these disturbing conditions and locate internal stillness amidst the chaos of our minds and the arena round us.

When we embark on the journey of Kriya Yoga, doubts might also additionally stand up, thinking the effectiveness of the exercising or our potential to collect the preferred results. These doubts can be disheartening and may prevent our improvement. However, it's miles crucial to don't forget that doubt is a natural part of the increase way. It is an invitation to dive deeper into our workout and explore the underlying motives of those doubts.

One way to navigate doubts is through self-reflected photo and introspection. Take the time to take a seat quietly and observe your thoughts and emotions. Are there any underlying fears or insecurities which are fueling your doubts? By acknowledging and addressing the ones fears, we're capable of begin to get to the bottom of the layers of resistance and flow into within the course of an area of more clarity and accept as real with.

Another powerful device is to are trying to find steering from a certified trainer or mentor. They can provide precious insights and assist, assisting us navigate the traumatic situations and doubts that stand up on our spiritual adventure. Engaging in regular satsangs or spiritual gatherings can also create a experience of community and help, reminding us that we are not on my own in our struggles.

Inner resistance is each different obstacle that often arises ultimately of the workout of Kriya

Yoga. It manifests as a reluctance to take a seat for meditation, a restlessness within the mind, or a regular circulate of distractions. This resistance can be tough to overcome, but with staying strength and perseverance, it could be converted proper right into a profound possibility for growth.

One way to cope with internal resistance is thru gentle place and dedication to our exercise. Creating a normal everyday and sticking to it, irrespective of the internal resistance, can assist installation a basis of balance and popularity. Additionally, incorporating different yogic practices inclusive of asanas (physical postures) and pranayama (respiratory wearing occasions) can help calm the thoughts and put together it for meditation.